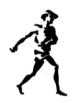

Stan Lee Presents
THE MIGHTY MARVEL STRENGTH AND FITNESS BOOK

Written by ANN PICARDO
Illustrated by JOE GIELLA

SIMON AND SCHUSTER · NEW YORK

Published by Simon and Schuster
A Gulf+Western Company
Rockefeller Center, 630 Fifth Avenue
New York, New York 10020

Manufactured in the United States of America

1   2   3   4   5   6   7   8   9   10

Library of Congress Cataloging in Publication Data

Lee, Stan.
   Stan Lee presents The Mighty Marvel strength
and fitness book.

   1. Exercise — Pictorial works. I. Picardo, Ann.
II. Giella, Joe. III. Title: The Mighty Marvel
strength and fitness book.
RA78I.L46 1976   613.7'1   76-14486

ISBN 0-671-22312-7

Contents

Foreword

Exercise is of paramount importance in enjoying good health, regardless of what age you are.

Today we know that obesity leads to poor health. Not only is diet important, but exercise also plays a very singular role in physical fitness. One of the toughest exercises (which The Invisible Girl forgot to mention in her part of the book) is to push yourself away from the dinner table.

It has been demonstrated by scientific studies that strenuous exercise releases a substance into your blood that reduces your appetite. If you exercise just before your main meal of the day, whether it is at noontime or at night, your desire to eat will be lessened and you will be satisfied to eat less. Fat people, heed and take notice!

As you perform the exercises you'll be learning in this book, the health you will be gaining can someday make you a superhero!

Alvin Robert Mintz, M.D.
Morristown, New Jersey
Fellow of the American Academy
of Pediatrics
Clinical Assistant Professor of
Pediatrics, New Jersey College
of Medicine and Dentistry

Introduction

This is not going to be a heavy-handed exercise book. In fact, it's not even going to be a heavy exercise book — maybe a pound and a half tops. So even if you're low on muscles, you'll be able to hoist this book up to eye level and start yourself on a fitness program, Marvel-made-to-order.

Even though we'll be cracking jokes and punning puns and alliterating alliterations just like in the comic books, don't let our lighthearted manner fool you. We'll be showing you some terrific exercises and giving you a lot of information about what you can do to make yourself healthier. If you snicker a small snicker every so often, so much the better.

There are no horribly demanding exercises in the book, but to make sure you don't leap into an exercise that's too tough, start at the beginning and work your way through.

If along the way you find any of the exercises difficult for you, leave them for a while (while you write us a nasty letter) and go back to them in a week or so.

It's also a good idea to take it easy the first time you try a new exercise, and as a general rule, it's better to exercise twenty or thirty minutes a day instead of saving it all up and killing yourself for two hours once a week.

So take a deep breath, Marvelites, and get at it!

A.P.

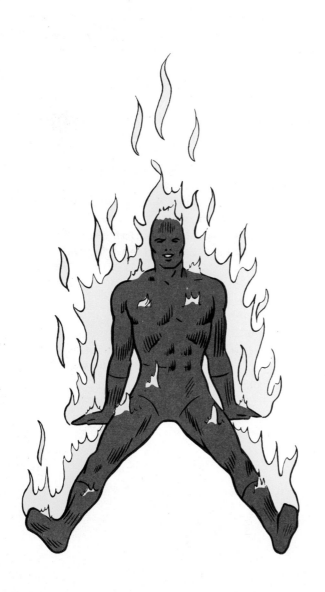

THE HEAT'S ON:
Warm-Up Exercises by
The Human Torch

Gangway! In this chapter, everybody's favorite Fahrenheiter will help you with exercises that make special use of his supertalents.

In oncoming chapters a lot of Torchie's friends (and a few of his enemies) will be teaching you exercises they're especially suited for. But if you hotfooted it into their exercises with cold muscles (not to mention cold feet) you could really hurt yourself, and we wouldn't want that to happen to the likes of you.

Warm-ups are a MUST before engaging in any strenuous physical activity. You don't have to kill yourself spending a lot of time on each exercise; just do each one a few times and move on to the next.

So turn the page, faithful ones, and FLAME ON!

The Torchie Twist

STAND ON YOUR RIGHT FOOT
AND TURN THE HEEL OF YOUR
WRONG FOOT (SOMETIMES
KNOWN AS YOUR LEFT FOOT)
OUT AS FAR AS YOU CAN.

1

THE BUMP
WAS NEVER
LIKE THIS!

2

THEN TURN YOUR LEFT
HEEL IN AS FAR AS
POSSIBLE.

3 SWITCH FEET AND START
ALL OVER. DO A HALF
DOZEN WITH EACH FOOT
AND THEN DO A HALF
DOZEN AT TWICE THE
SPEED. (LIKE A 33⅓
RECORD PLAYED AT 45!)

14

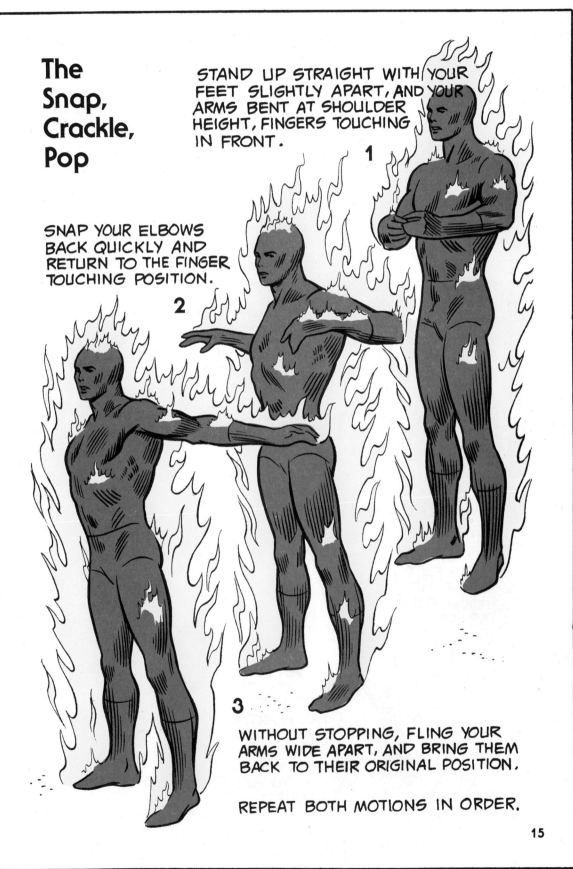

The Snap, Crackle, Pop

STAND UP STRAIGHT WITH YOUR FEET SLIGHTLY APART, AND YOUR ARMS BENT AT SHOULDER HEIGHT, FINGERS TOUCHING IN FRONT.

1

SNAP YOUR ELBOWS BACK QUICKLY AND RETURN TO THE FINGER TOUCHING POSITION.

2

3

WITHOUT STOPPING, FLING YOUR ARMS WIDE APART, AND BRING THEM BACK TO THEIR ORIGINAL POSITION.

REPEAT BOTH MOTIONS IN ORDER.

15

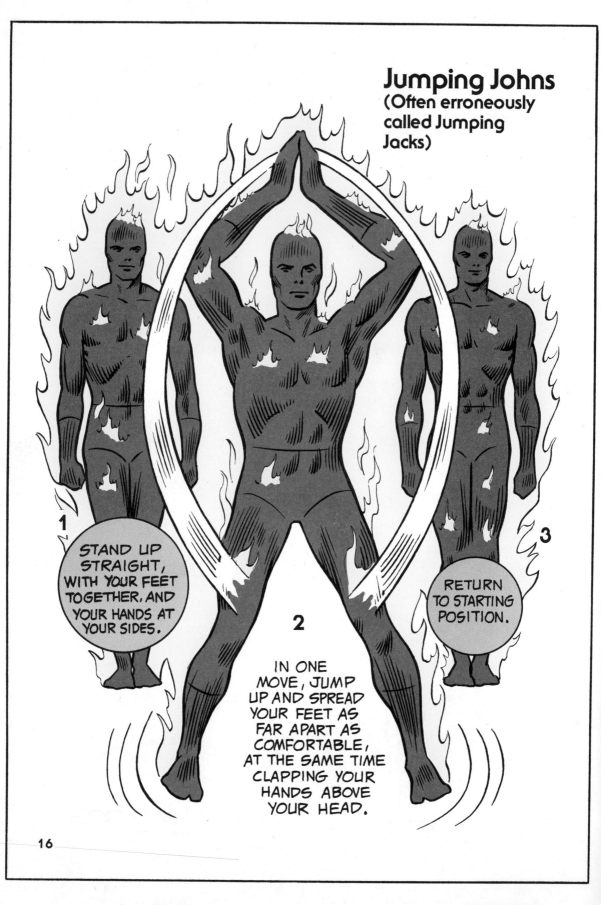

The Johnny Storm Stroll

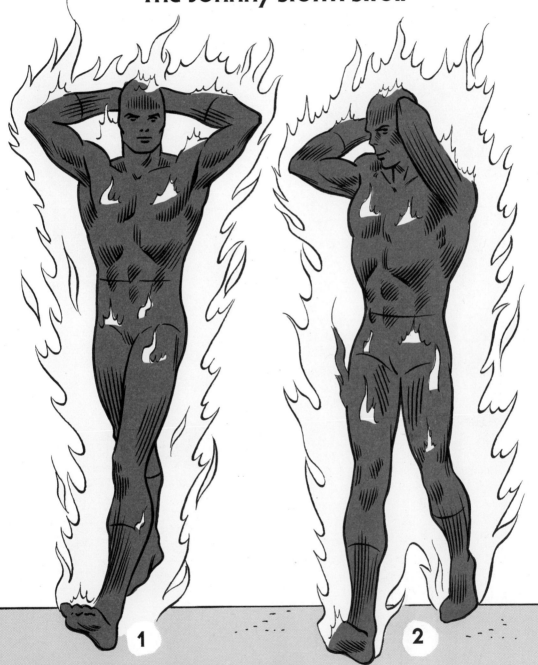

1

JOIN YOUR HANDS BEHIND YOUR HEAD AND BEGIN TO WALK FORWARD WITH LONG STEPS. (YOU MAY NEED TO MOVE OUTDOORS FOR THIS UNLESS YOU LIVE ABOVE A BOWLING ALLEY.)

2

AS YOU WALK, TWIST YOUR BODY TO THE SAME SIDE AS YOUR FORWARD LEG.

Torch's Take-Off Stretch

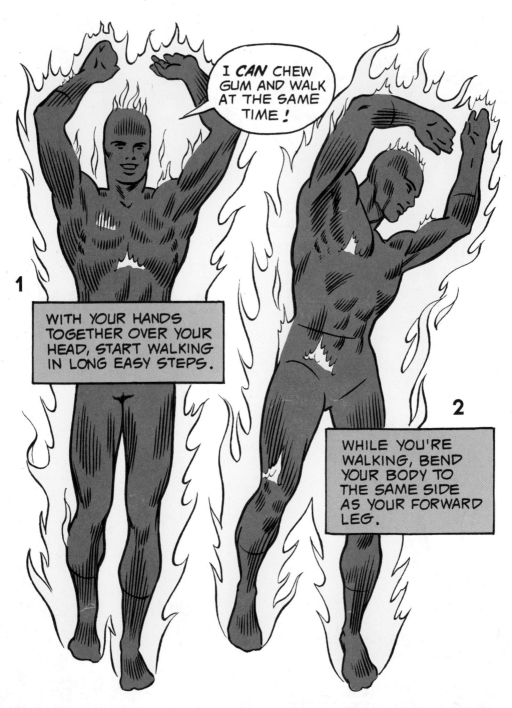

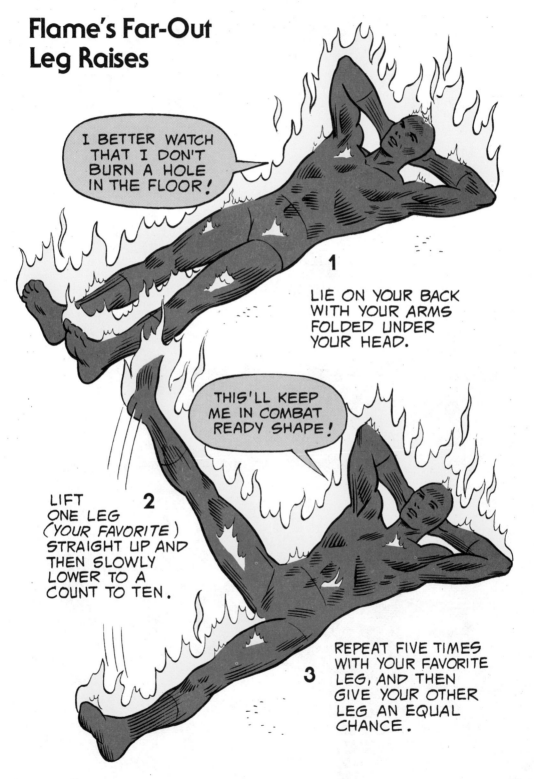

19

Torchie's Tendinous Tummy Tilt

1 LIE FLAT ON YOUR STOMACH, HANDS AT YOUR SIDES.

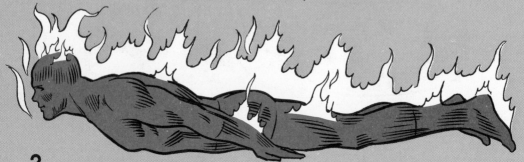

2 SLOWLY LIFT YOUR HEAD AS FAR OFF THE FLOOR AS POSSIBLE,

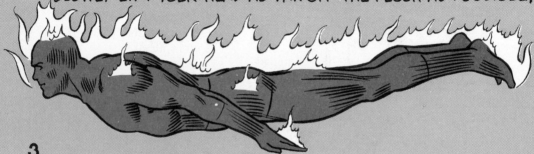

3 THEN RAISE YOUR LEGS UP AS HIGH AS YOU CAN.

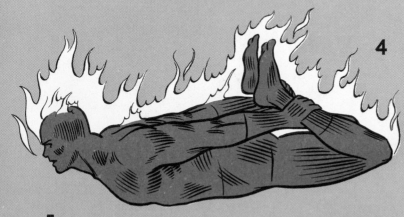

4 COMPLAIN TO YOURSELF A LITTLE AND THEN BEND YOUR KNEES, GRABBING YOUR ANKLES WITH YOUR HANDS. (IF YOU CAN.)

5 THEN, YOU'LL BE HAPPY TO HEAR, YOU CAN RELAX. (YOU'LL NEED IT AT FIRST. BUT AFTER YOU GET GOOD AT THIS, YOU'LL EVEN BE ABLE TO ROCK BACK AND FORTH ON YOUR STOMACH.)

Johnny's Juxtaposed Toe Touches

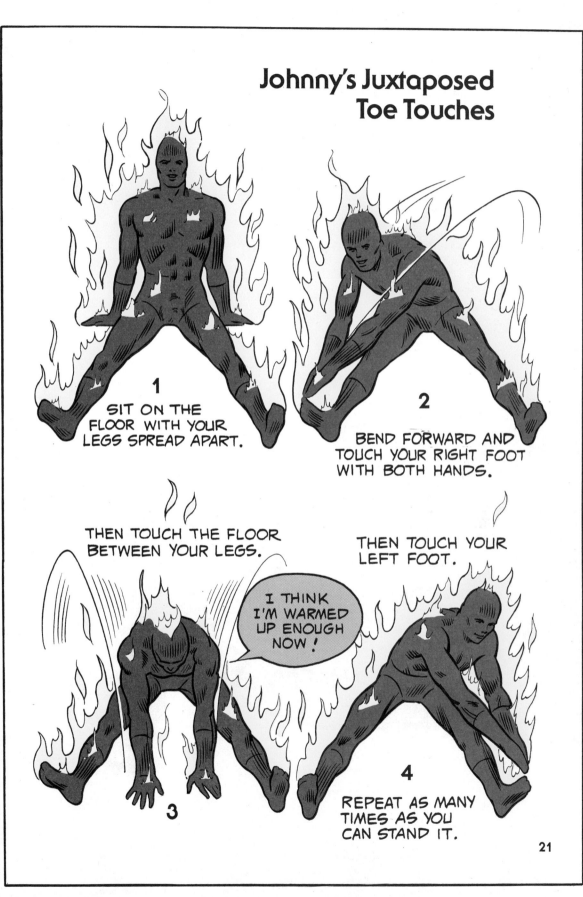

1 SIT ON THE FLOOR WITH YOUR LEGS SPREAD APART.

2 BEND FORWARD AND TOUCH YOUR RIGHT FOOT WITH BOTH HANDS.

THEN TOUCH THE FLOOR BETWEEN YOUR LEGS.

THEN TOUCH YOUR LEFT FOOT.

I THINK I'M WARMED UP ENOUGH NOW!

3

4 REPEAT AS MANY TIMES AS YOU CAN STAND IT.

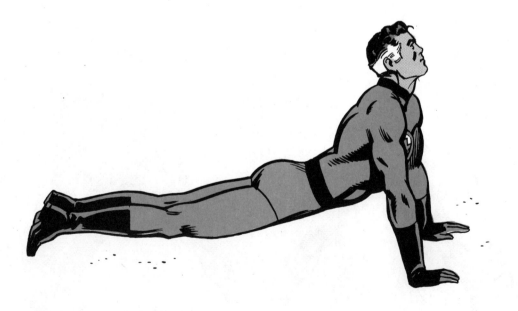

YOU CAN GET THERE FROM HERE:

2

Stretching Exercises from
Mr. Fantastic

One of the best things about stretching exercises is that they make you feel so good. And what's more, for those of us with a tendency to get older every day or so, stretching exercises can limber us, relax us and keep us from feeling our age.

To wit (not to mention forsooth and anon), you never see Reed Richards struggling to keep up with his precocious partners, and we hate to mention this, Reed, but you are getting a little gray at the temples.

For Reed's not-so-secret secrets, READ ON!

Reed's Upwardly Mobile Back and Stomach Stretch

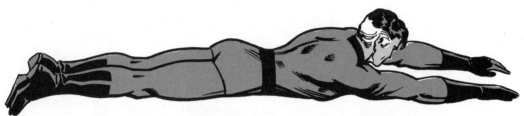

1 LIE FLAT ON THE FLOOR, ON YOUR STOMACH WITH YOUR ARMS IN FRONT OF YOU.

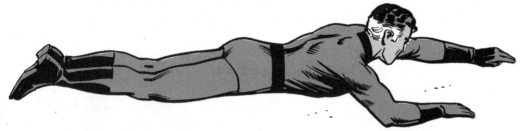

2 MOVE YOUR RIGHT HAND BACK A COUPLE OF INCHES, THEN MOVE YOUR LEFT HAND BACK AN EQUAL DISTANCE.

3 KEEP DOING THIS UNTIL YOUR ARMS ARE STRAIGHT, AND YOUR HEAD IS HIGH.

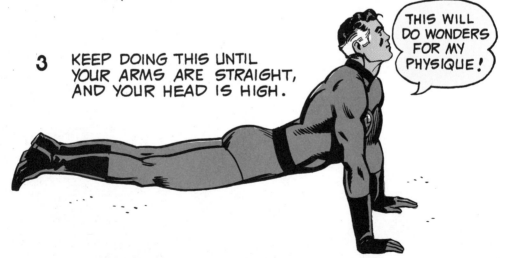

4 RETURN TO YOUR ORIGINAL POSITION AND REPEAT.

Stretcho's Super Sit-Up

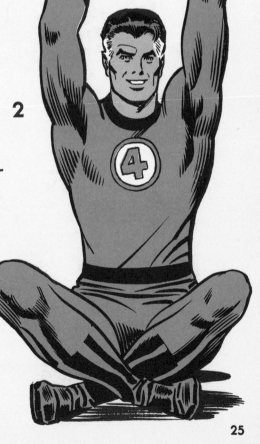

1 SIT UP ON THE FLOOR, WITH YOUR LEGS CROSSED *AMERICAN* INDIAN STYLE (*OUR LITTLE TRIBUTE TO THE BICENTENNIAL*) AND YOUR HANDS AT YOUR SIDES.

2

ONE AT A TIME, PUT YOUR HANDS WAY ABOVE YOUR HEAD, AND REACH AND PULL AS HIGH AS YOU CAN, STRAIGHTENING YOUR BACK. DON'T WIGGLE YOUR BODY, JUST PULL WITH YOUR ARMS.

3

RELAX AND START OVER.

Mr. Fantastic's Noble Knee and Thigh Stretch

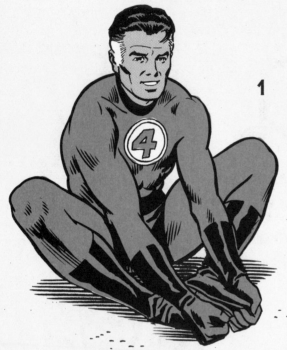

1

SIT ERECT (OR, IF YOU PREFER, SIT UP STRAIGHT), WITH THE BOTTOMS OF YOUR FEET TOGETHER. CLASP YOUR HANDS AROUND YOUR FEET, AND BRING YOUR FEET AS CLOSE TO YOUR BODY AS POSSIBLE.

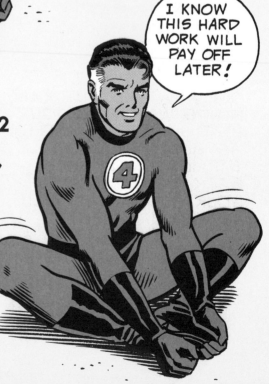

I KNOW THIS HARD WORK WILL PAY OFF LATER!

2

PULL UP ON YOUR FEET SO THAT YOUR KNEES BEND TOWARD THE FLOOR AS FAR AS THEY CAN.

3

HOLD THIS POSITION WHILE YOU COUNT TO TEN. RELAX FOR A FEW SECONDS AND REPEAT.

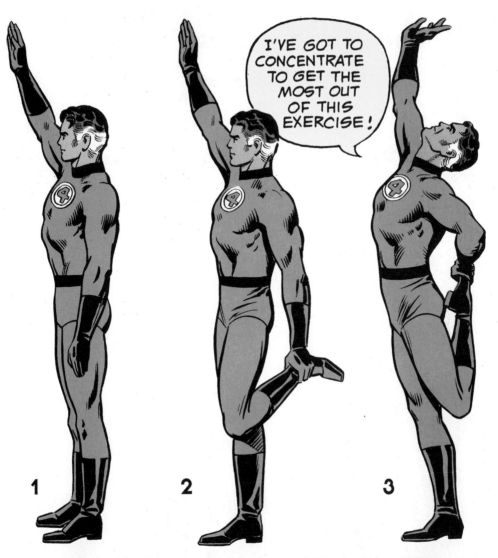

Reed's Righteous and Responsible Arm and Leg Lift

1 STAND UP STRAIGHT AND RAISE YOUR RIGHT ARM OVER YOUR HEAD.

2 SLOWLY LIFT YOUR LEFT LEG BEHIND YOU AND HOLD IT WITH YOUR LEFT HAND. (USE YOUR RIGHT HAND FOR BALANCE SO IT WON'T FEEL LEFT OUT...OR RIGHT OUT, AS THE CASE MAY BE.)

3 SLOWLY (HAVE YOU NOTICED THAT EXERCISE BOOKS NEVER TELL YOU TO DO ANYTHING QUICKLY?) REACH BACK WITH YOUR RIGHT ARM AND LIFT YOUR LEFT FOOT UP AS FAR AS YOU CAN. WITH YOUR HEAD DROPPED BACK, HOLD STILL FOR A FEW SECONDS.

RELAX AND REPEAT WITH YOUR OPPOSITE HAND AND FOOT.

Rubberlegs' Prestigious Pole Hang

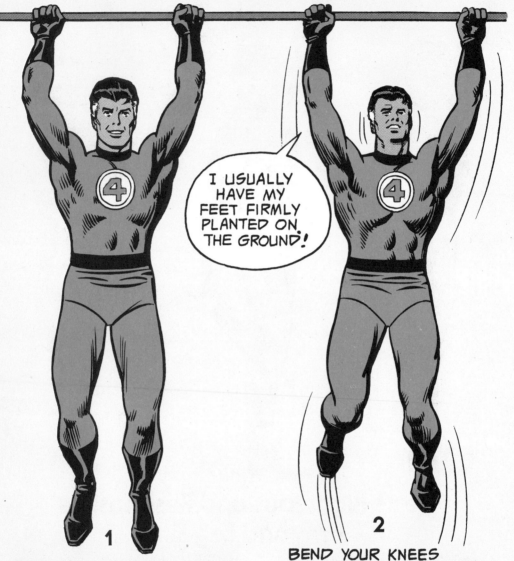

I USUALLY HAVE MY FEET FIRMLY PLANTED ON THE GROUND!

1

FIND A PRESTIGIOUS POLE WHICH IS JUST ABOVE YOUR REACH. (IF YOU CAN'T FIND A PRESTIGIOUS POLE, YOU CAN SETTLE FOR A PLEBEIAN POLE — WE'LL JUST CHANGE THE NAME OF THE EXERCISE.)

GRAB HOLD OF IT WITH BOTH YOUR HANDS.

2

BEND YOUR KNEES BEHIND YOU, AND HANG FOR A COUNT OF TEN (OR, SIMPLY "HANG TEN" AS THE SILVER SURFER MIGHT SAY).

THEN, *BEFORE* YOU LET GO WITH YOUR HANDS, PUT YOUR FEET ON THE FLOOR. (DID WE REALLY THINK YOU WERE *THAT* DUMB ?)

Reed's Rotating Toe Touches

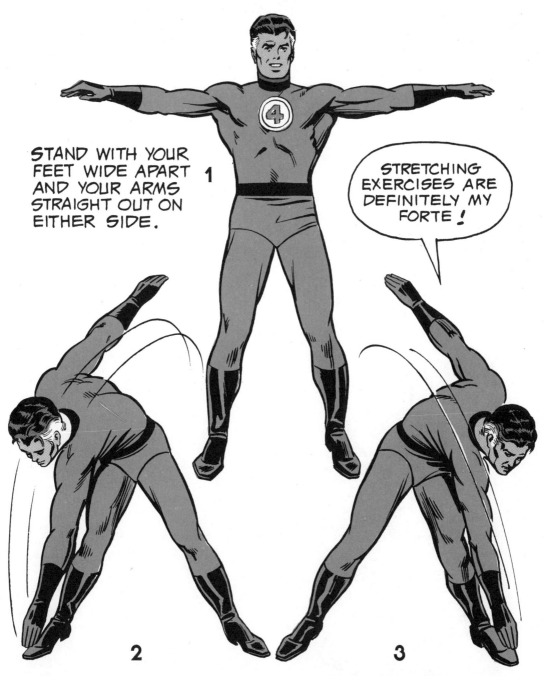

STAND WITH YOUR FEET WIDE APART AND YOUR ARMS STRAIGHT OUT ON EITHER SIDE.

1

STRETCHING EXERCISES ARE DEFINITELY MY FORTE!

2

BEND DOWN AND TOUCH YOUR RIGHT TOE WITH YOUR LEFT HAND.

3

STAND UP AGAIN AND TOUCH YOUR LEFT TOE WITH YOUR RIGHT HAND.

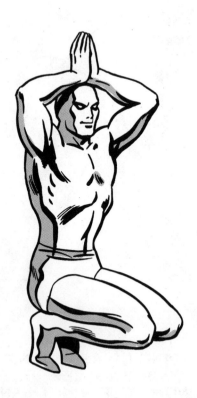

THE STRAIGHT AND NARROW:

3

Posture and Balance Exercises from
The Silver Surfer

Anyone who has been hanging ten through the solar system for an eon or two knows all too well the importance of good posture and balance.

But aside from helping you look good on a surfboard (or even on a date, for that matter), correct posture lets all parts of your body work like they are supposed to work ... without being cramped or pushed around by spines that aren't lined up the way they're supposed to be lined up and so forth. (Gee, was _that_ a long sentence. Glad my gnarly old English teacher isn't going to be reading this!)

Good balance and good posture go together like Sue Storm and Reed Richards ... and if you do all the exercises in this chapter you can have both — good posture and good balance, that is. If you want Sue and Reed, you'll just have to fork over twenty-five cents for the next issue of <u>The Fantastic Four</u>.

Herald's Honorific Head Turns

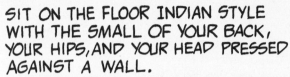

1 SIT ON THE FLOOR INDIAN STYLE WITH THE SMALL OF YOUR BACK, YOUR HIPS, AND YOUR HEAD PRESSED AGAINST A WALL.

YOUR HANDS SHOULD BE ON THE FLOOR BESIDE YOU WITH YOUR PALMS TURNED UP, AND YOU SHOULD PULL YOUR SHOULDERS BACK TOWARD THE WALL AND DOWN.

IF THIS ISN'T ENOUGH TO REMEMBER, YOUR HEAD SHOULD BE HELD STRAIGHT AND PUSHED UP TOWARD THE CEILING, TOO.

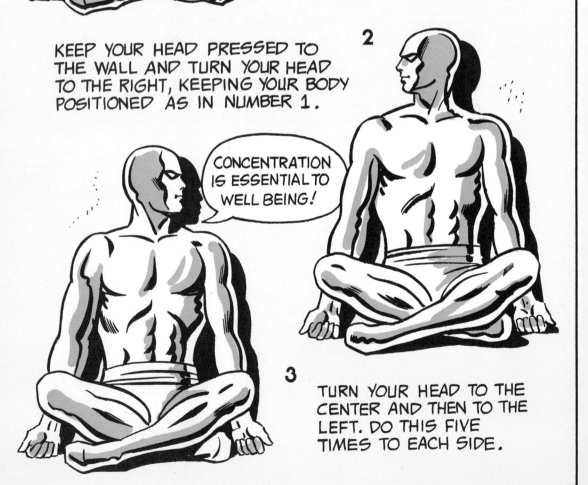

KEEP YOUR HEAD PRESSED TO THE WALL AND TURN YOUR HEAD TO THE RIGHT, KEEPING YOUR BODY POSITIONED AS IN NUMBER 1.

2

CONCENTRATION IS ESSENTIAL TO WELL BEING!

3

TURN YOUR HEAD TO THE CENTER AND THEN TO THE LEFT. DO THIS FIVE TIMES TO EACH SIDE.

Solid Sterling's Back Perfectors

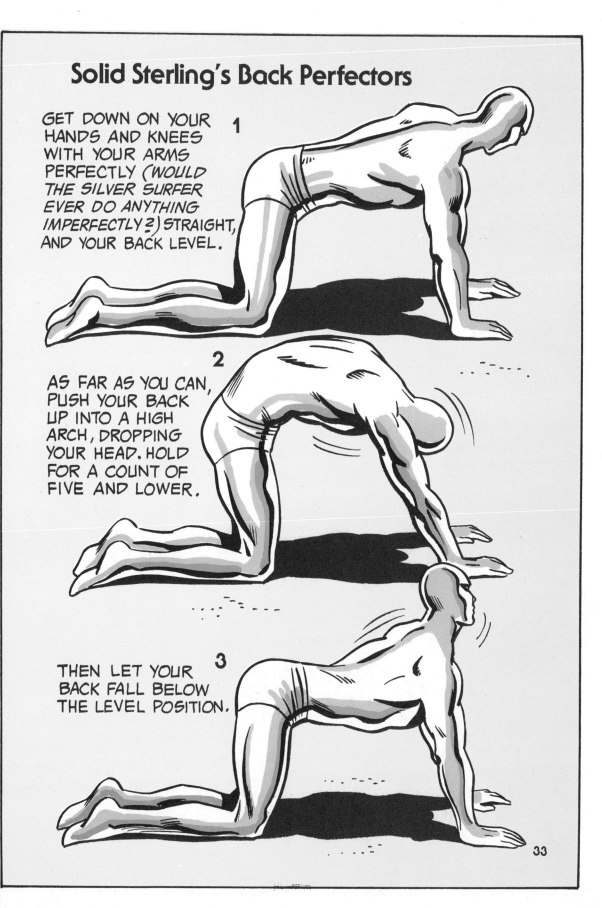

GET DOWN ON YOUR HANDS AND KNEES WITH YOUR ARMS PERFECTLY *(WOULD THE SILVER SURFER EVER DO ANYTHING IMPERFECTLY?)* STRAIGHT, AND YOUR BACK LEVEL. **1**

2 AS FAR AS YOU CAN, PUSH YOUR BACK UP INTO A HIGH ARCH, DROPPING YOUR HEAD. HOLD FOR A COUNT OF FIVE AND LOWER.

3 THEN LET YOUR BACK FALL BELOW THE LEVEL POSITION.

Silver Surfer's Heralded Highwires

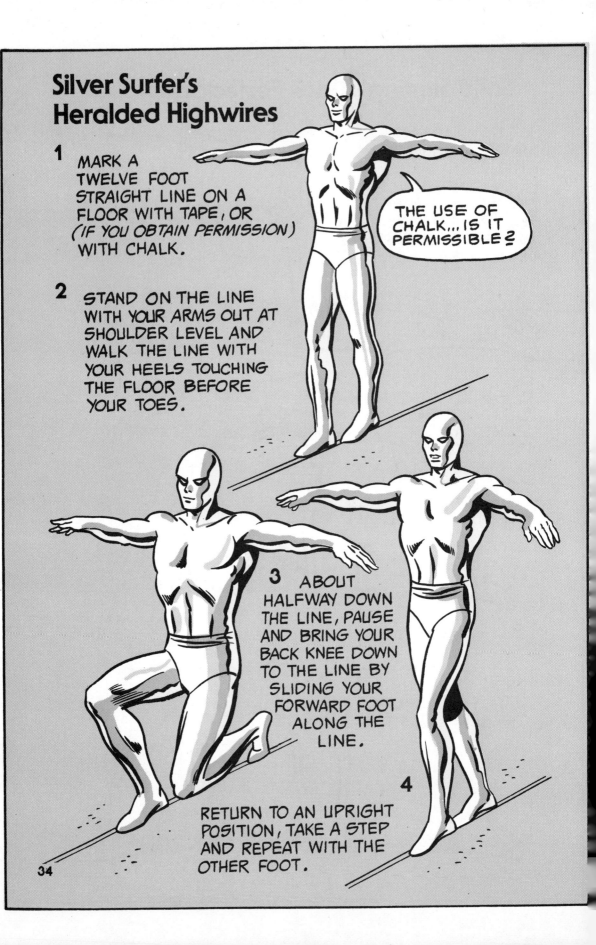

1 MARK A TWELVE FOOT STRAIGHT LINE ON A FLOOR WITH TAPE, OR (IF YOU OBTAIN PERMISSION) WITH CHALK.

THE USE OF CHALK... IS IT PERMISSIBLE?

2 STAND ON THE LINE WITH YOUR ARMS OUT AT SHOULDER LEVEL AND WALK THE LINE WITH YOUR HEELS TOUCHING THE FLOOR BEFORE YOUR TOES.

3 ABOUT HALFWAY DOWN THE LINE, PAUSE AND BRING YOUR BACK KNEE DOWN TO THE LINE BY SLIDING YOUR FORWARD FOOT ALONG THE LINE.

4 RETURN TO AN UPRIGHT POSITION, TAKE A STEP AND REPEAT WITH THE OTHER FOOT.

34

The Galactus Grip

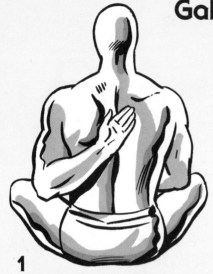

1

SIT INDIAN STYLE ON THE FLOOR AND BRING YOUR LEFT ARM UP LIKE YOU SEE IN THE PICTURE.

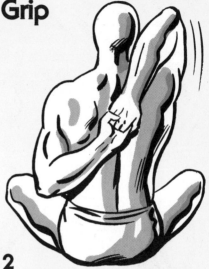

2

BRING YOUR RIGHT HAND OVER YOUR SHOULDER AND GRASP YOUR LEFT HAND.

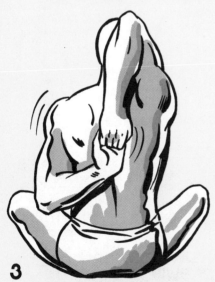

3

PULL *DOWN* WITH YOUR LEFT HAND AND HOLD FOR A COUNT OF FIVE.

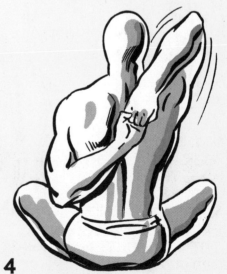

4

PULL *UP* WITH YOUR RIGHT HAND AND HOLD FOR A COUNT OF FIVE.

DO THIS SIX TIMES THIS WAY AND THEN DO IT ANOTHER SIX TIMES SWITCHING YOUR ARMS AROUND TO THE OTHER SIDE.

The Tireless Toe Twist

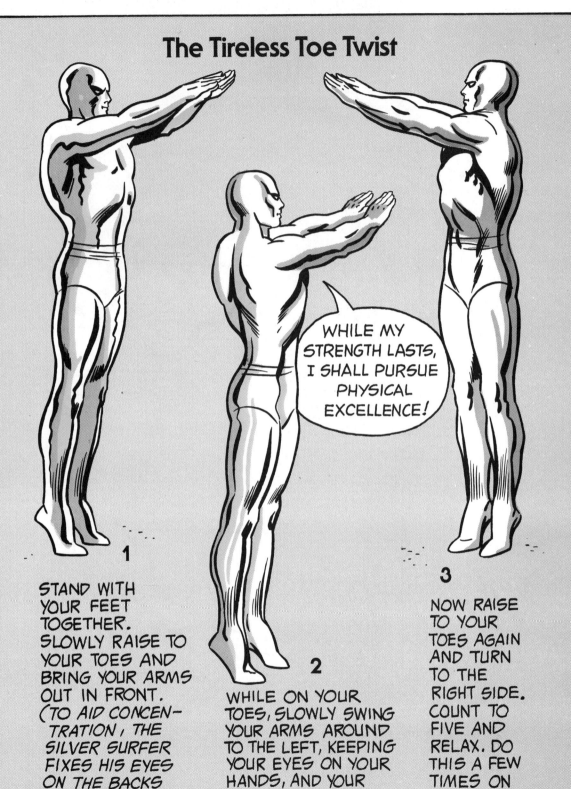

WHILE MY STRENGTH LASTS, I SHALL PURSUE PHYSICAL EXCELLENCE!

1
STAND WITH YOUR FEET TOGETHER. SLOWLY RAISE TO YOUR TOES AND BRING YOUR ARMS OUT IN FRONT. (TO AID CONCEN- TRATION, THE SILVER SURFER FIXES HIS EYES ON THE BACKS OF HIS HANDS.)

2
WHILE ON YOUR TOES, SLOWLY SWING YOUR ARMS AROUND TO THE LEFT, KEEPING YOUR EYES ON YOUR HANDS, AND YOUR FEET IN THE SAME POSITION. REMAIN FOR A COUNT OF FIVE.

3
NOW RAISE TO YOUR TOES AGAIN AND TURN TO THE RIGHT SIDE. COUNT TO FIVE AND RELAX. DO THIS A FEW TIMES ON EACH SIDE.

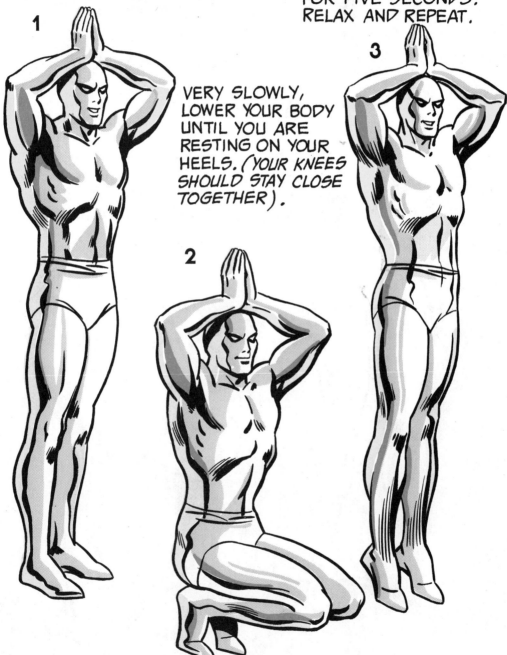

STAND WITH THE PALMS OF YOUR HANDS PRESSED TOGETHER AND HELD ON YOUR HEAD.

1

SMOOTHLY RAISE UP UNTIL YOU ARE STANDING ON YOUR TOES. HOLD FOR FIVE SECONDS. RELAX AND REPEAT.

3

VERY SLOWLY, LOWER YOUR BODY UNTIL YOU ARE RESTING ON YOUR HEELS. (YOUR KNEES SHOULD STAY CLOSE TOGETHER).

2

Surfer's Solar System Stances

The Interplanetary Leap

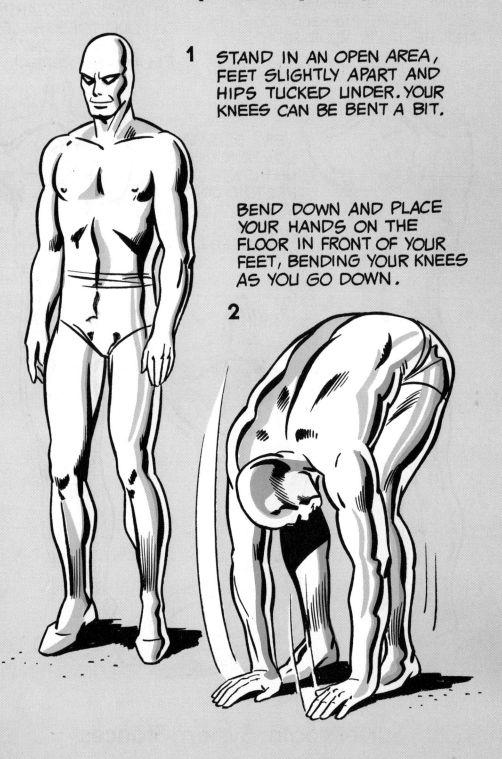

1 STAND IN AN OPEN AREA, FEET SLIGHTLY APART AND HIPS TUCKED UNDER. YOUR KNEES CAN BE BENT A BIT.

BEND DOWN AND PLACE YOUR HANDS ON THE FLOOR IN FRONT OF YOUR FEET, BENDING YOUR KNEES AS YOU GO DOWN.

2

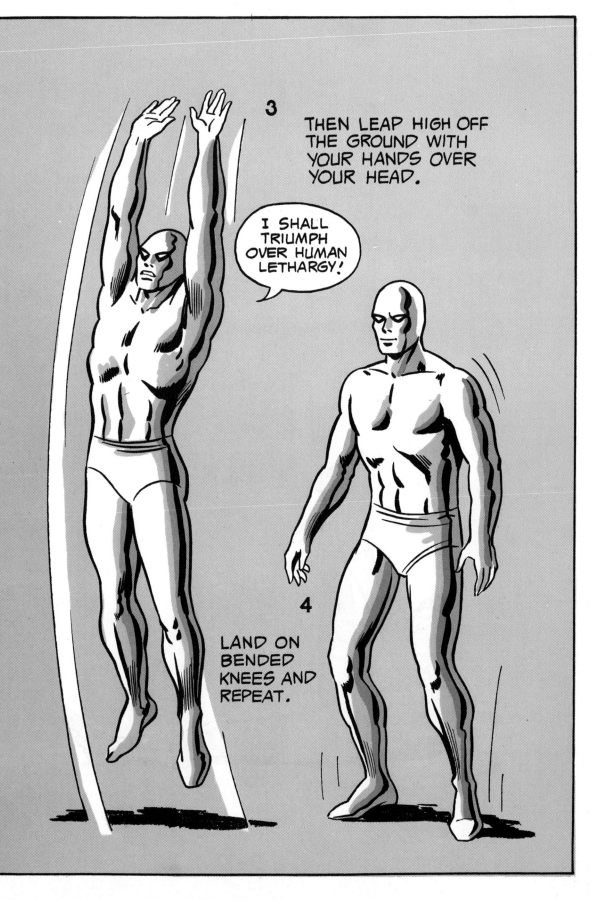

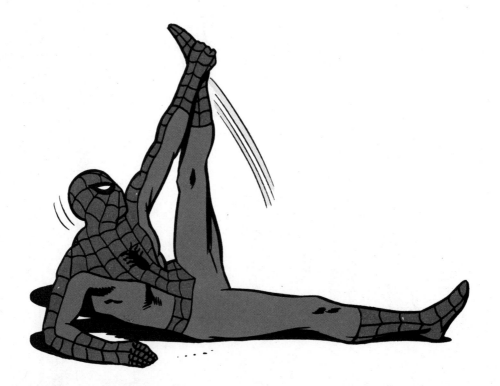

YOU CAN'T KEEP A GOOD MAN DOWN:

4

Agility and Climbing Tips from Everybody's Favorite Wall Crawler

No book would be complete without some words from everybody's favorite Webhead. In fact, he has such a way with words that he was talking about strength and fitness a long time before Simon and Schuster ever thought of this book. (Actually, Stan Lee and some clever New York literary agent thought of this book, but we'll let Simon and Schuster take the credit. After all, it's their money.)

At any rate, getting back to the Webhead, way back in the swingin' sixties Spider-Man was heard to say, "No matter who you are, there's always someone stronger."

Now, personally, we don't think this quote can hold a candle to "With great power... etc.," but who are we to judge?

But anyway, be that as it Aunt May, Spidey's contribution to our treatise on fitness and health is contained in the following exercises designed to limber you up.

So without further ado, as they say in those Las Vegas lounges ... "Here he is, ladies and gentlemen, the Amazing Spider-Man!"

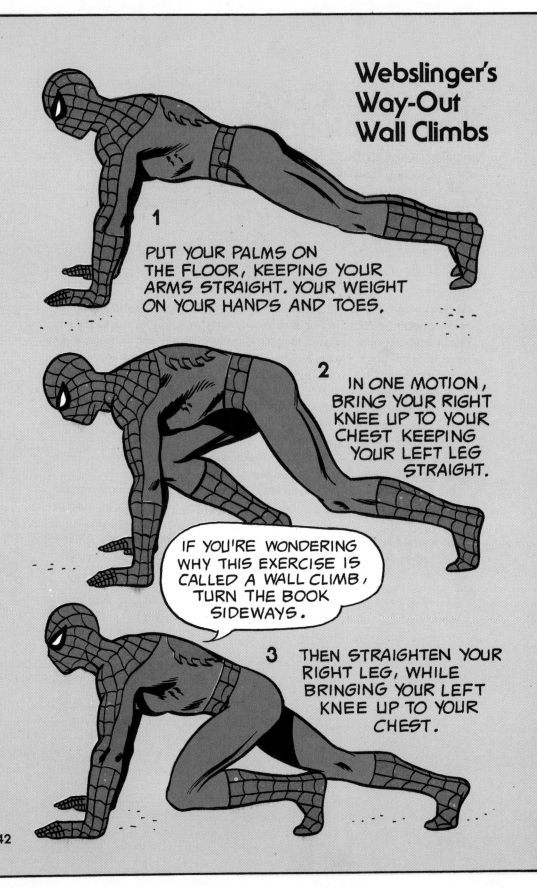

Webslinger's Way-Out Wall Climbs

1 PUT YOUR PALMS ON THE FLOOR, KEEPING YOUR ARMS STRAIGHT. YOUR WEIGHT ON YOUR HANDS AND TOES,

2 IN ONE MOTION, BRING YOUR RIGHT KNEE UP TO YOUR CHEST KEEPING YOUR LEFT LEG STRAIGHT.

IF YOU'RE WONDERING WHY THIS EXERCISE IS CALLED A WALL CLIMB, TURN THE BOOK SIDEWAYS.

3 THEN STRAIGHTEN YOUR RIGHT LEG, WHILE BRINGING YOUR LEFT KNEE UP TO YOUR CHEST.

Spidey's Supple Sidewinders

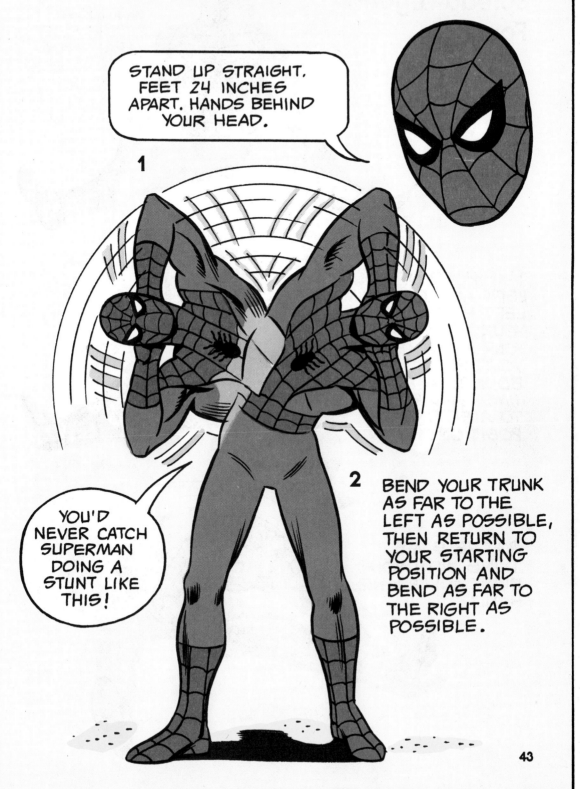

STAND UP STRAIGHT, FEET 24 INCHES APART. HANDS BEHIND YOUR HEAD.

1

YOU'D NEVER CATCH SUPERMAN DOING A STUNT LIKE THIS!

2 BEND YOUR TRUNK AS FAR TO THE LEFT AS POSSIBLE, THEN RETURN TO YOUR STARTING POSITION AND BEND AS FAR TO THE RIGHT AS POSSIBLE.

Spindlemann's Spread-Legged Foot Pull

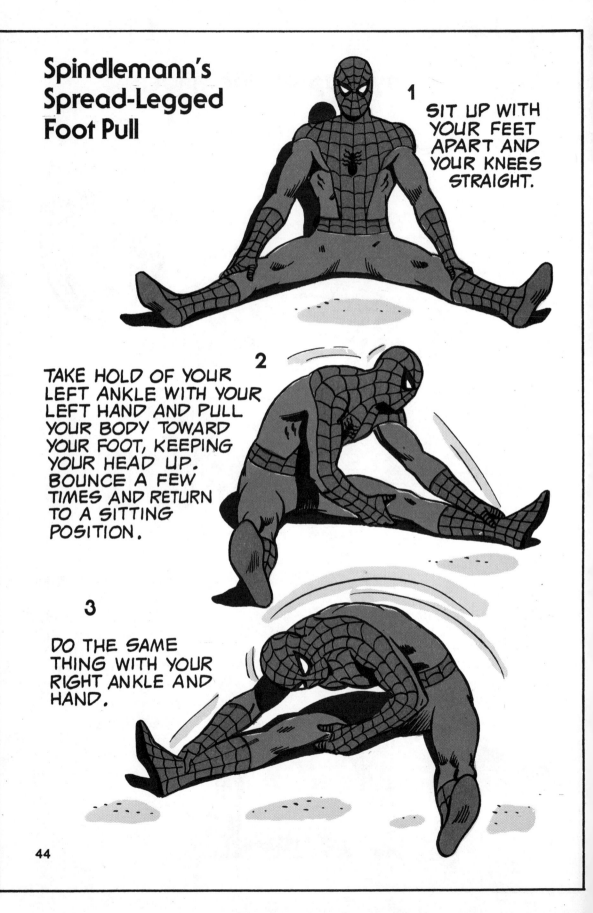

1 SIT UP WITH YOUR FEET APART AND YOUR KNEES STRAIGHT.

2 TAKE HOLD OF YOUR LEFT ANKLE WITH YOUR LEFT HAND AND PULL YOUR BODY TOWARD YOUR FOOT, KEEPING YOUR HEAD UP. BOUNCE A FEW TIMES AND RETURN TO A SITTING POSITION.

3 DO THE SAME THING WITH YOUR RIGHT ANKLE AND HAND.

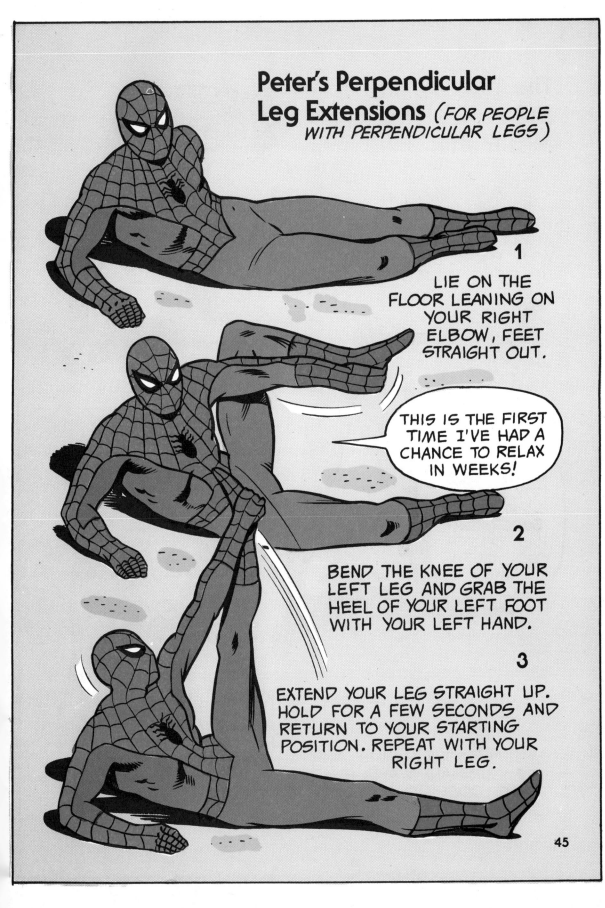

The
Little
Miss Muffet

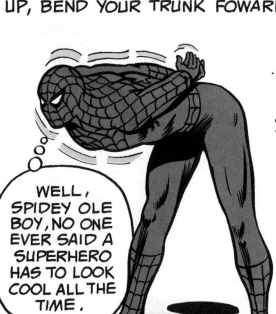

1

STAND WITH YOUR FEET SPREAD APART, YOUR HANDS JOINED BEHIND YOUR BACK. KEEPING YOUR HEAD UP, BEND YOUR TRUNK FOWARD.

WELL, SPIDEY OLE BOY, NO ONE EVER SAID A SUPERHERO HAS TO LOOK COOL ALL THE TIME.

2

BOUNCE YOUR BODY UP AND DOWN A HALF DOZEN TIMES.

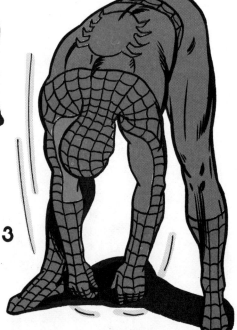

3

UNCLASP YOUR HANDS, AND LET YOUR HANDS AND HEAD HANG LOOSE TO A COUNT OF EIGHT.

The Spider Bounce

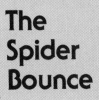

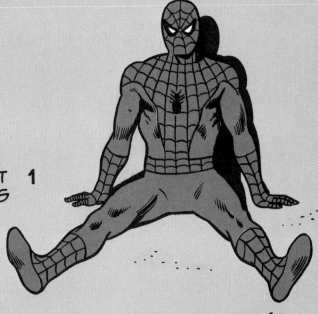

SIT UP STRAIGHT **1**
WITH YOUR LEGS
SPREAD APART.

2 EASE YOURSELF DOWN TO A LYING POSITION (*BUT ALWAYS TELL THE TRUTH*) WITH YOUR HANDS OVER YOUR HEAD.

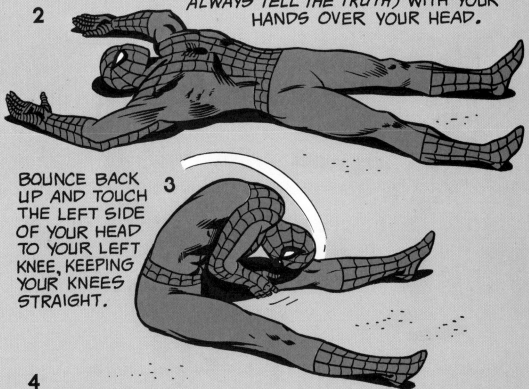

BOUNCE BACK **3**
UP AND TOUCH
THE LEFT SIDE
OF YOUR HEAD
TO YOUR LEFT
KNEE, KEEPING
YOUR KNEES
STRAIGHT.

4

RETURN TO YOUR STARTING POSITION, AND REPEAT
WITH YOUR RIGHT LEG.

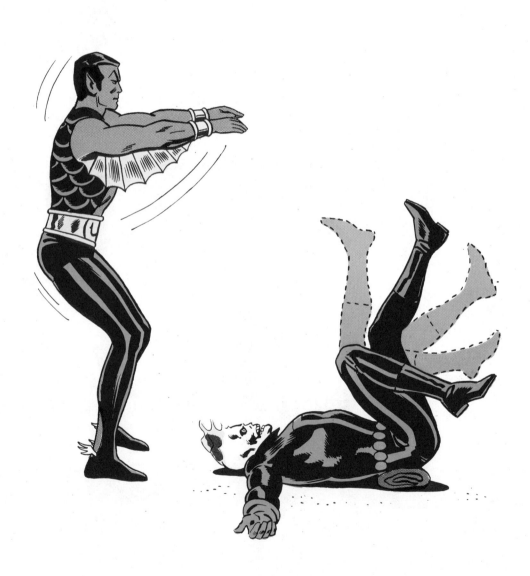

EVERYBODY LOVES A GOOD SPORT:

5

Swimming and Bike-Riding Exercises from That Doubtful Duo, Sub-Mariner and Ghost Rider

As the Olympic Committee sometimes says, "Sports is the international language." (Some people might prefer that they say "Sports are the international language," but all of us grammarians know they'd be dead wrong.)

Well, if sports can bring people who speak different languages together, is it too much to hope that sports could unite two people as different as Subby and Ghost Rider? Certainly not! Through the magic of Marvel, we've done it. What does logic have to do with comic books anyway?

As everyone knows, those summertime favorites swimming and bicycling require a little conditioning, especially if you've been hanging out around the television all winter, complaining of fatigue when you had to get up to change the channel.

Well, our two dynamic divergents here have just what you need to get back in shape ... so climb into your swim or sweat suit and get going!

Namor's Nimble-Footed Flutters

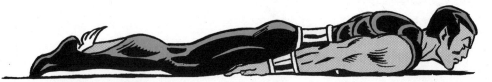

1 LIE ON THE FLOOR ON YOUR STOMACH, WITH YOUR HANDS PALMS DOWN.

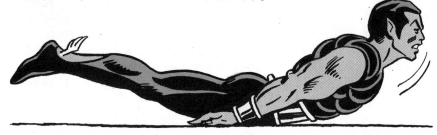

2 ARCH YOUR BACK SO THAT YOUR CHEST AND LEGS ARE RAISED.

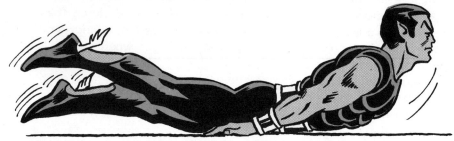

3 KEEPING YOUR LEGS STRAIGHT BUT LOOSE, DO A FLUTTER KICK.

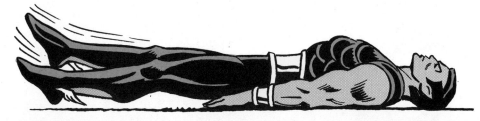

4 NOW FLIP OVER ON YOUR BACK (*WE COULD HAVE SAID "TURN" OVER ON YOUR BACK" BUT WE WANTED TO KEEP TO A NAUTICAL THEME*) AND DO THE SAME WITH YOUR LEGS.

Pointy Ears' Partial Knee Bends

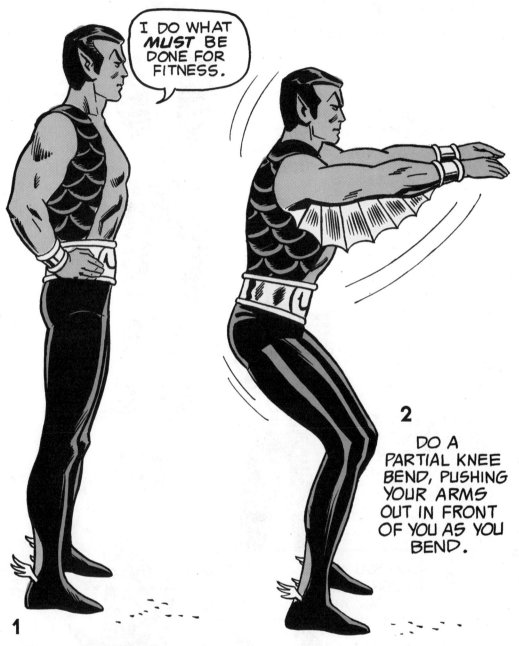

1

STAND UP STRAIGHT (YOU'D THINK WE EXPECTED YOU TO STAND UP CROOKED!) WITH YOUR HANDS ON YOUR HIPS.

2

DO A PARTIAL KNEE BEND, PUSHING YOUR ARMS OUT IN FRONT OF YOU AS YOU BEND.

3

RETURN TO YOUR ORIGINAL STANCE AND REPEAT.

The Avenging Son's Arm Strengtheners

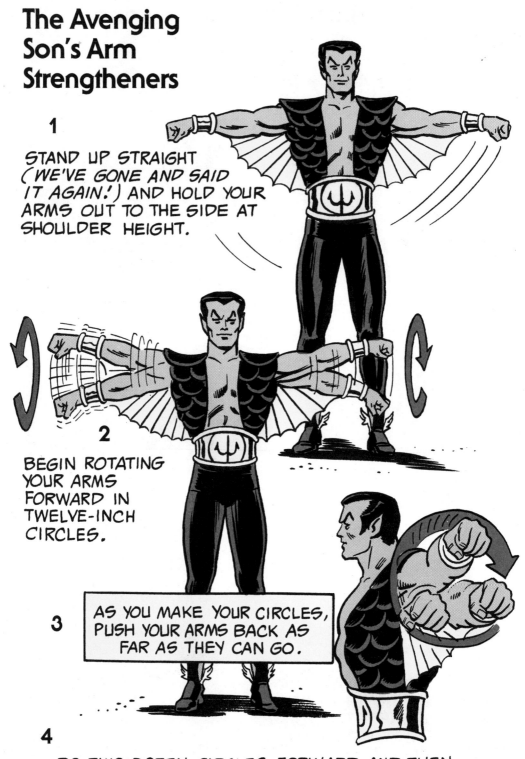

1

STAND UP STRAIGHT (WE'VE GONE AND SAID IT AGAIN!) AND HOLD YOUR ARMS OUT TO THE SIDE AT SHOULDER HEIGHT.

2

BEGIN ROTATING YOUR ARMS FORWARD IN TWELVE-INCH CIRCLES.

3

AS YOU MAKE YOUR CIRCLES, PUSH YOUR ARMS BACK AS FAR AS THEY CAN GO.

4

DO TWO DOZEN CIRCLES FORWARD AND THEN TWO DOZEN BACKWARD.

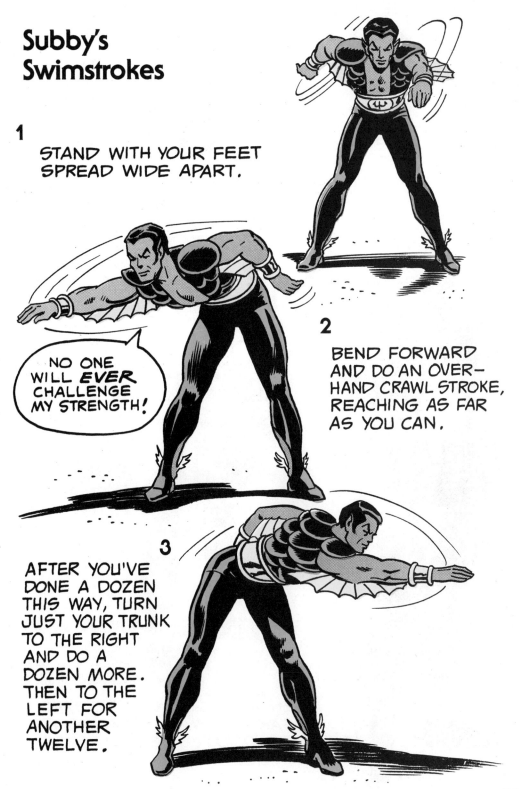

Subby's Swimstrokes

1

STAND WITH YOUR FEET SPREAD WIDE APART.

NO ONE WILL *EVER* CHALLENGE MY STRENGTH!

2

BEND FORWARD AND DO AN OVER-HAND CRAWL STROKE, REACHING AS FAR AS YOU CAN.

3

AFTER YOU'VE DONE A DOZEN THIS WAY, TURN JUST YOUR TRUNK TO THE RIGHT AND DO A DOZEN MORE. THEN TO THE LEFT FOR ANOTHER TWELVE.

Subby's Backward Swimstrokes
(OFTTIMES CALLED THE BACKSTROKE)

STAND UP STRAIGHT WITH YOUR RIGHT ARM AT YOUR SIDE AND THE BACK OF YOUR LEFT HAND AGAINST YOUR CHEEK. PUSH YOUR ELBOW BACK AS FAR AS YOU CAN.

1

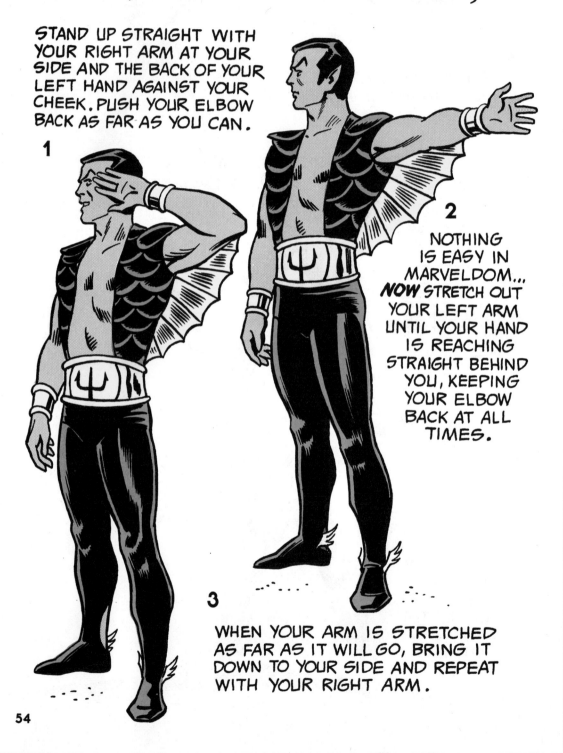

2

NOTHING IS EASY IN MARVELDOM... *NOW* STRETCH OUT YOUR LEFT ARM UNTIL YOUR HAND IS REACHING STRAIGHT BEHIND YOU, KEEPING YOUR ELBOW BACK AT ALL TIMES.

3

WHEN YOUR ARM IS STRETCHED AS FAR AS IT WILL GO, BRING IT DOWN TO YOUR SIDE AND REPEAT WITH YOUR RIGHT ARM.

Ghost Rider's Bizarre Bicycles

LIE DOWN ON THE FLOOR,
FACE AND KNEES UP WITH
YOUR ARMS STRAIGHT
OUT AND EVEN YOUR
PALMS FACING UP.

1

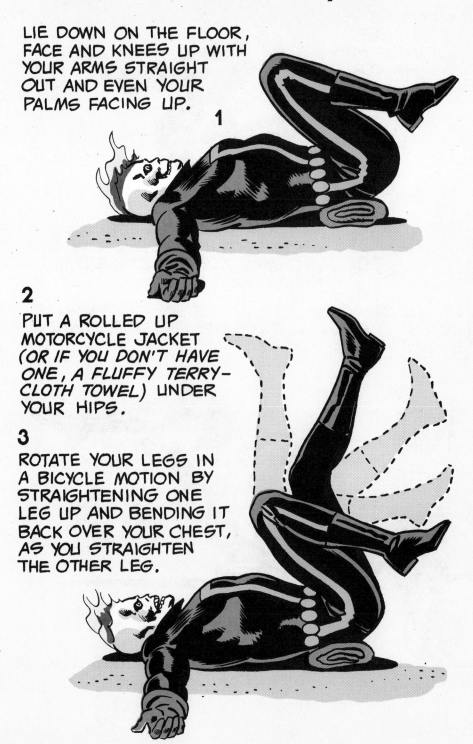

2

PUT A ROLLED UP
MOTORCYCLE JACKET
(OR IF YOU DON'T HAVE
ONE, A FLUFFY TERRY-
CLOTH TOWEL) UNDER
YOUR HIPS.

3

ROTATE YOUR LEGS IN
A BICYCLE MOTION BY
STRAIGHTENING ONE
LEG UP AND BENDING IT
BACK OVER YOUR CHEST,
AS YOU STRAIGHTEN
THE OTHER LEG.

Ghost Rider's Even Bizarrer Backward Bicycles

LIE DOWN ON THE FLOOR, FACE UP AND KNEES UP WITH YOUR ARMS STRAIGHT OUT AND EVEN YOUR PALMS FACING UP.

1

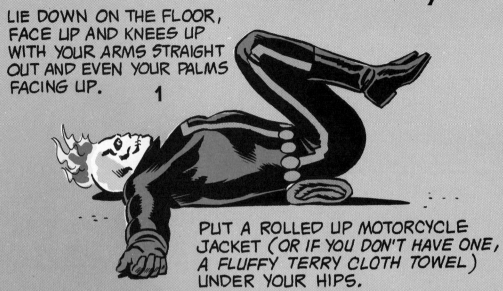

PUT A ROLLED UP MOTORCYCLE JACKET (OR IF YOU DON'T HAVE ONE, A FLUFFY TERRY CLOTH TOWEL) UNDER YOUR HIPS.

(WHO ARE WE TRYING TO KID... IF THIS SOUNDS FAMILIAR, IT'S BECAUSE IT'S EXACTLY THE SAME AS THE BEGINNING OF THE LAST MEMORABLE EXERCISE.)

NO USE JUST LYIN' HERE... I MIGHT AS WELL GET HEALTHIER!

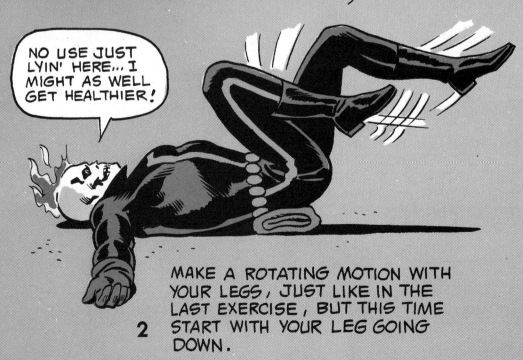

2 MAKE A ROTATING MOTION WITH YOUR LEGS, JUST LIKE IN THE LAST EXERCISE, BUT THIS TIME START WITH YOUR LEG GOING DOWN.

Skull Head's Soleus Stretch

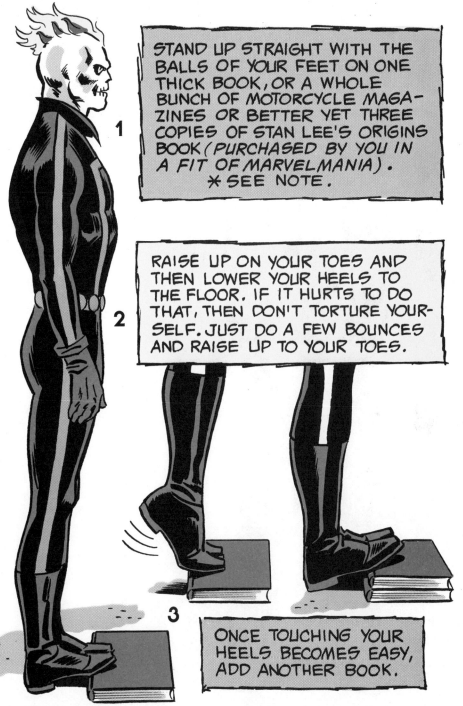

1 STAND UP STRAIGHT WITH THE BALLS OF YOUR FEET ON ONE THICK BOOK, OR A WHOLE BUNCH OF MOTORCYCLE MAGA-ZINES OR BETTER YET THREE COPIES OF STAN LEE'S ORIGINS BOOK (*PURCHASED BY YOU IN A FIT OF MARVELMANIA*).
✳ SEE NOTE.

2 RAISE UP ON YOUR TOES AND THEN LOWER YOUR HEELS TO THE FLOOR. IF IT HURTS TO DO THAT, THEN DON'T TORTURE YOUR-SELF. JUST DO A FEW BOUNCES AND RAISE UP TO YOUR TOES.

3 ONCE TOUCHING YOUR HEELS BECOMES EASY, ADD ANOTHER BOOK.

✳ ALL KIDDING ASIDE, A STURDY THICK BOOK IS THE SAFEST.

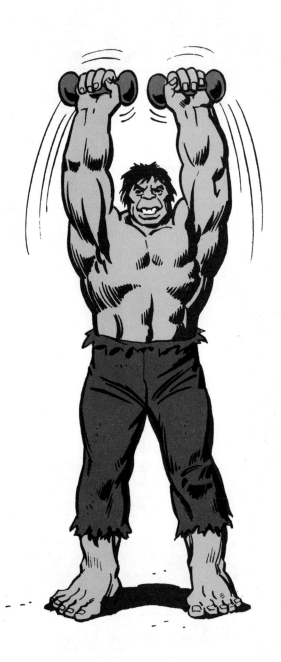

HOW TO MAKE THE KIDS AT THE BEACH GREEN WITH ENVY:

6

Body Builders from The
Incredible Hulk

Here comes The Incredible Hulk with a pulsating panorama of body builders designed to make you <u>almost</u> as powerful as our green giant ... but not quite. (We couldn't tell you all his secrets or you might go out and start a comic book of your own.)

With body builders you have to start small and work your way up to better feats (and hands) of daring. Even if you want to get into weight lifting in a big way, you should begin with a series of setting-up exercises, which happen, O Lucky Reader, to be pretty good body builders in themselves. (As a matter of fact, the first four exercises in this chapter are just what Doc Oc ordered.)

In case you aren't Jack La Lanne's long-lost nephew (or niece) and don't have a closet full of weights (or barbells as they used to call them when Hulk was still Bruce Banner), don't despair! Many people (and many people <u>with muscles</u> too) feel that the safest and most effective way to weight-train is to do a lot of lifting of little weights instead of a little lifting with heavier weights.

You can buy weight bags (one to three pounds) in a sporting-goods store, or you can start working out this minute with one-pound vegetable cans from your kitchen cupboard. As a special tribute to our isometric idol, you might choose the brand bearing his nefarious nickname ... No, we don't call him Del Monte!

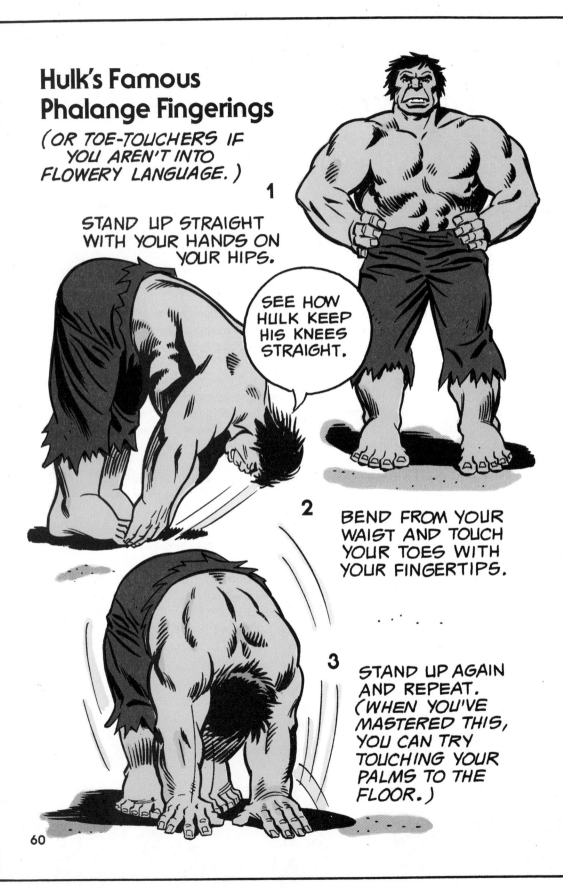

Hulk's Laudable Leg Levitations

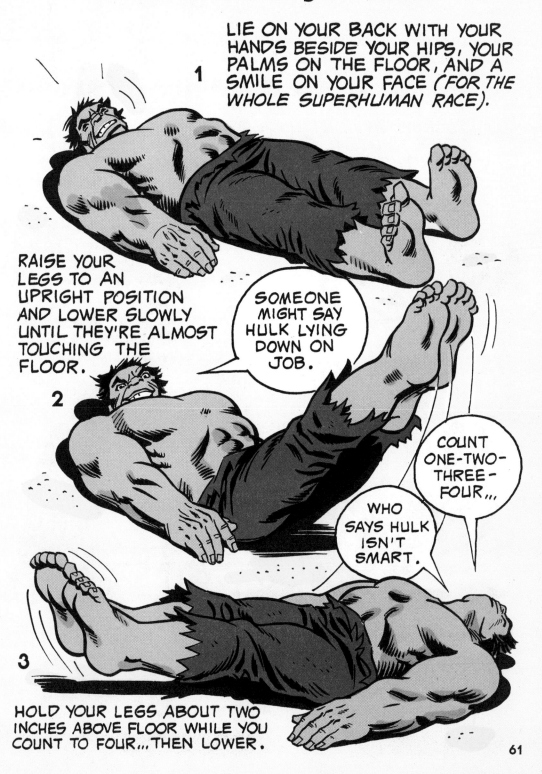

1 LIE ON YOUR BACK WITH YOUR HANDS BESIDE YOUR HIPS, YOUR PALMS ON THE FLOOR, AND A SMILE ON YOUR FACE (FOR THE WHOLE SUPERHUMAN RACE).

2 RAISE YOUR LEGS TO AN UPRIGHT POSITION AND LOWER SLOWLY UNTIL THEY'RE ALMOST TOUCHING THE FLOOR.

SOMEONE MIGHT SAY HULK LYING DOWN ON JOB.

COUNT ONE-TWO-THREE-FOUR...

WHO SAYS HULK ISN'T SMART.

3 HOLD YOUR LEGS ABOUT TWO INCHES ABOVE FLOOR WHILE YOU COUNT TO FOUR...THEN LOWER.

61

Jade-Jaws' Just-So Sit-Ups

1 LIE ON YOUR BACK AND GET A FRIEND (OR ARCH ENEMY) TO HOLD YOUR FEET. (IF YOU HAVE NEITHER FRIEND NOR FOE HANDY, YOU CAN TUCK YOUR FEET UNDER SOME NEUTRAL PIECE OF FURNITURE.)

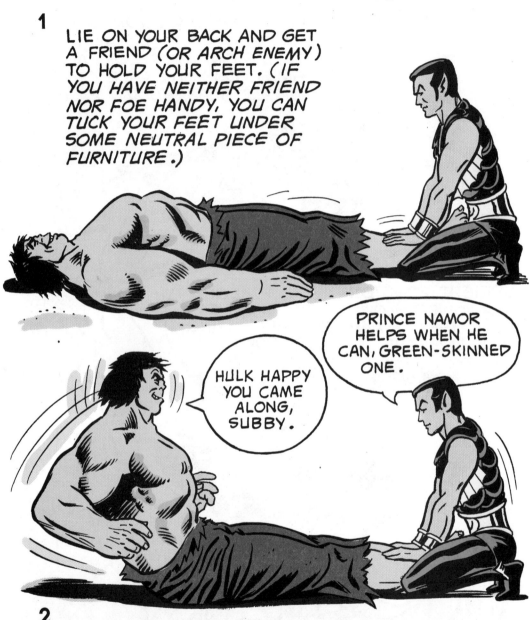

2 WITHOUT BENDING YOUR KNEES OR USING YOUR HANDS OR ARMS. RAISE UP TO A SITTING POSITION.

SLOWLY (SO YOU WON'T KNOCK YOURSELF OUT) **3** RETURN TO YOUR ORIGINAL POSITION.

Peagreen's Practical Push-Ups

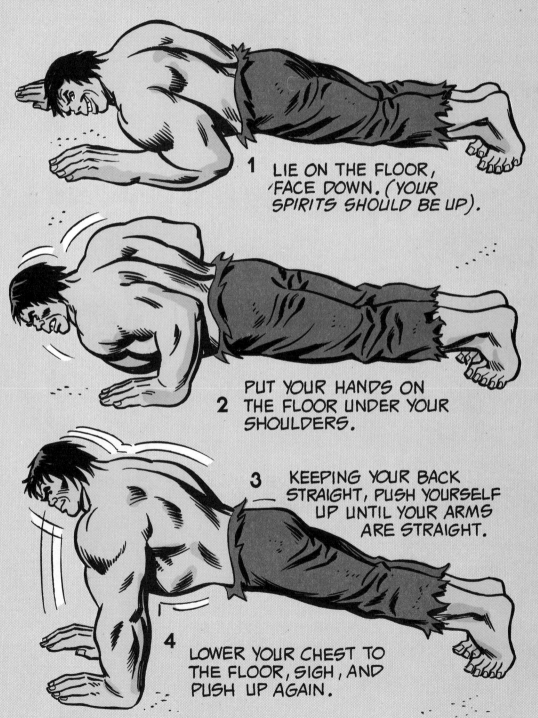

1 LIE ON THE FLOOR, FACE DOWN. (YOUR SPIRITS SHOULD BE UP).

2 PUT YOUR HANDS ON THE FLOOR UNDER YOUR SHOULDERS.

3 KEEPING YOUR BACK STRAIGHT, PUSH YOURSELF UP UNTIL YOUR ARMS ARE STRAIGHT.

4 LOWER YOUR CHEST TO THE FLOOR, SIGH, AND PUSH UP AGAIN.

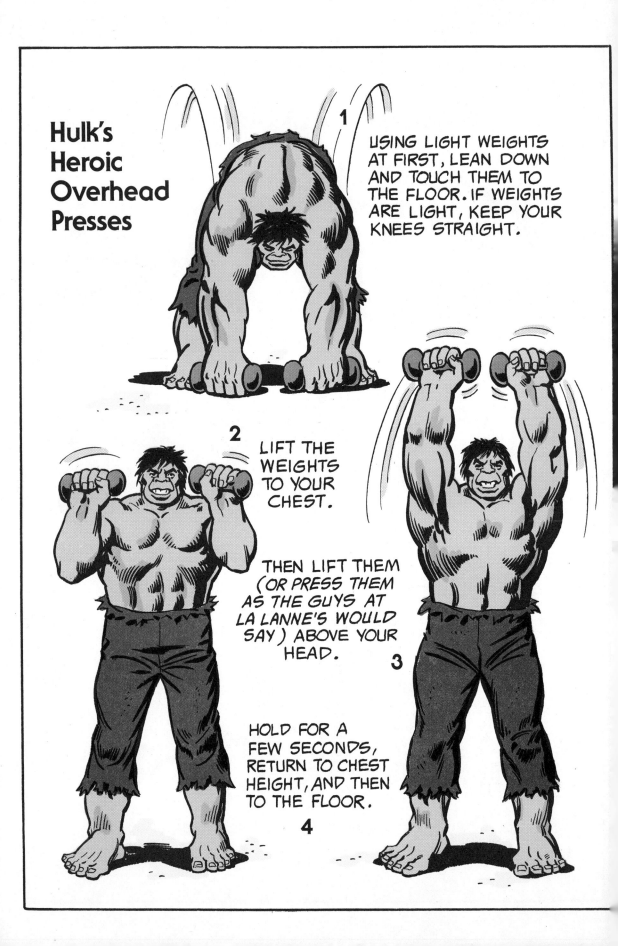

Hulk's Heroic Overhead Presses

1

USING LIGHT WEIGHTS AT FIRST, LEAN DOWN AND TOUCH THEM TO THE FLOOR. IF WEIGHTS ARE LIGHT, KEEP YOUR KNEES STRAIGHT.

2

LIFT THE WEIGHTS TO YOUR CHEST.

THEN LIFT THEM (OR PRESS THEM AS THE GUYS AT LA LANNE'S WOULD SAY) ABOVE YOUR HEAD.

3

HOLD FOR A FEW SECONDS, RETURN TO CHEST HEIGHT, AND THEN TO THE FLOOR.

4

Banner's Bellicose Bench Presses
(without a bench)*

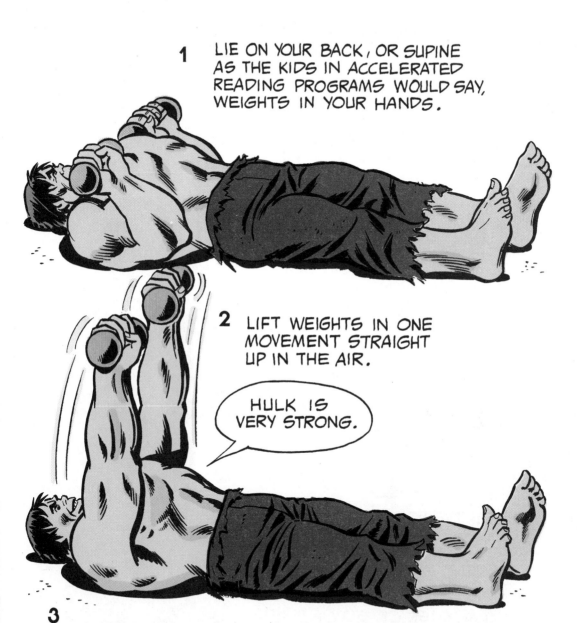

1 LIE ON YOUR BACK, OR SUPINE AS THE KIDS IN ACCELERATED READING PROGRAMS WOULD SAY, WEIGHTS IN YOUR HANDS.

2 LIFT WEIGHTS IN ONE MOVEMENT STRAIGHT UP IN THE AIR.

HULK IS VERY STRONG.

3 STRETCH YOUR ARMS HIGH, AND RETURN TO ORIGINAL POSITION. DO THIS A DOZEN OR SO TIMES, OR UNTIL YOUR ARMS ASK (NOT BEG) FOR MERCY.

✱ SEE HOW EASY WE'RE MAKING THIS FOR YOU?

The Incredible Curl

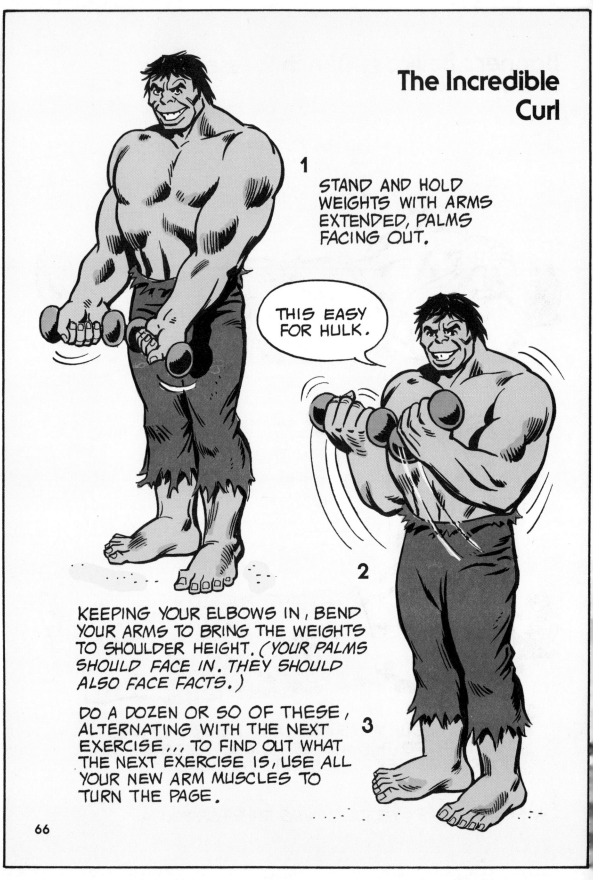

1

STAND AND HOLD
WEIGHTS WITH ARMS
EXTENDED, PALMS
FACING OUT.

THIS EASY
FOR HULK.

2

KEEPING YOUR ELBOWS IN, BEND
YOUR ARMS TO BRING THE WEIGHTS
TO SHOULDER HEIGHT. (YOUR PALMS
SHOULD FACE IN. THEY SHOULD
ALSO FACE FACTS.)

DO A DOZEN OR SO OF THESE,
ALTERNATING WITH THE NEXT
EXERCISE... TO FIND OUT WHAT
THE NEXT EXERCISE IS, USE ALL
YOUR NEW ARM MUSCLES TO
TURN THE PAGE.

3

The Incredible Uncurl

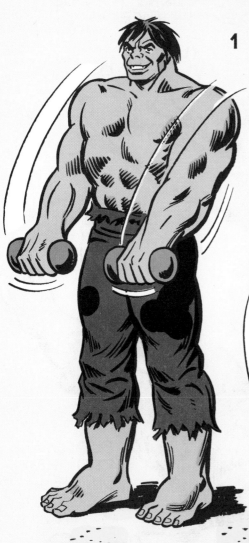

1

STAND AND HOLD WEIGHTS WITH ARMS EXTENDED, PALMS FACING IN.

KEEPING YOUR ELBOWS IN, BEND YOUR ARMS TO SHOULDER HEIGHT. (YOUR PALMS SHOULD BE FACING OUT.)

2

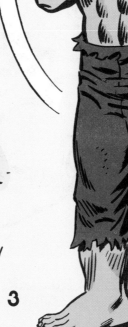

ALTERNATE WITH THE EXERCISE YOU HAVE FRESH IN YOUR MEMORY FROM THE LAST PAGE.

3

Jolly Green's Lateral Extensions

1 LIE ON YOUR BACK WITH YOUR ARMS HOLDING WEIGHTS STRAIGHT ABOVE YOUR FACE.

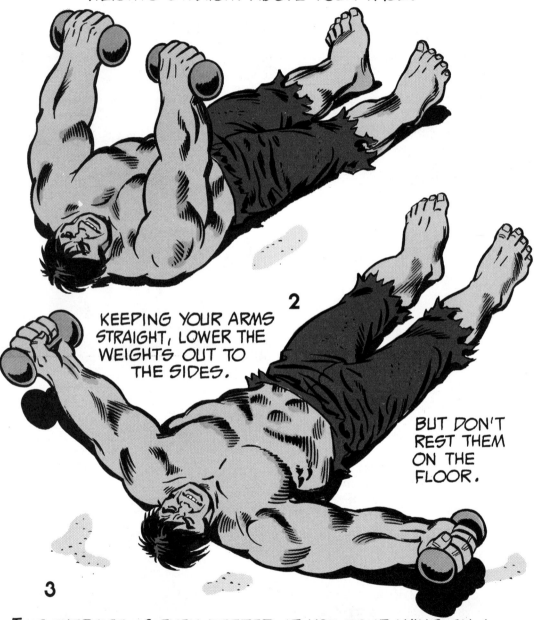

2 KEEPING YOUR ARMS STRAIGHT, LOWER THE WEIGHTS OUT TO THE SIDES.

BUT DON'T REST THEM ON THE FLOOR.

3 THIS EXERCISE IS EVEN BETTER, IF YOU DO IT LYING ON A BENCH... (LIKE THE ONE WE SAID YOU *DIDN'T* NEED BEFORE...)

REPEAT THIS MOTION A DOZEN OR SO TIMES.

Green Goliath's Odious Overhead Extensions

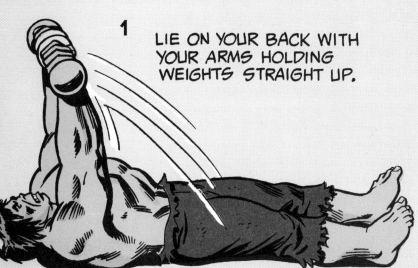

1 LIE ON YOUR BACK WITH YOUR ARMS HOLDING WEIGHTS STRAIGHT UP.

LOWER YOUR ARMS OVER YOUR HEAD, BUT DON'T REST THEM ON THE FLOOR. *(THAT WOULD BE TOO EASY.)*

2

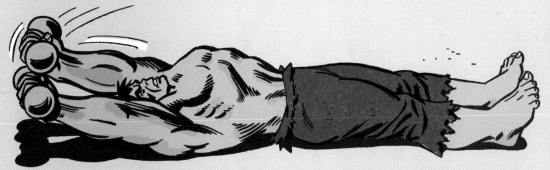

RETURN YOUR ARMS TO THE STRAIGHT UP POSITION AND THEN LOWER THEM FORWARD, BUT DON'T REST THEM ON YOUR THIGHS.

3

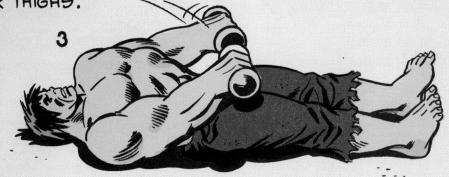

(ABOUT A DOZEN OF THESE SHOULD BE ENOUGH FOR ANY LARGE, GREEN PERSON.)

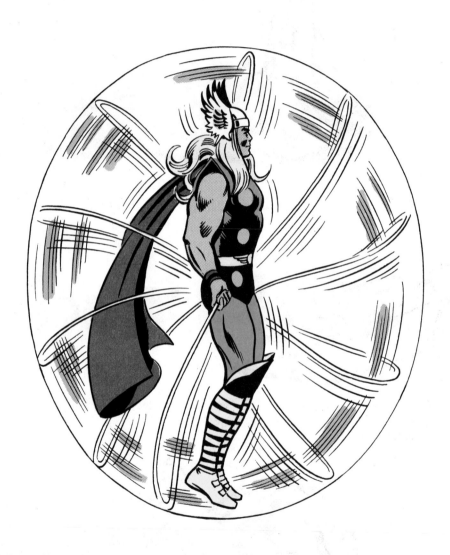

THIS NINE-POUND HAMMER IS A LITTLE TOO HEAVY:
Strength and Endurance Exercises from Thor

7

If ever someone looked in the bloom of health, it's our pal Goldilocks. How did he get that way? You guessed it! He's been exercising for years.

If you think it's easy lugging that hammer around all day, you'd better think again! It takes a lot of strength and stamina ... something Thor knows plenty about.

When we let him sneak a blue-eyed peek at this book, he insisted that he be allowed to share some of his favorite exercises with you.

So hold on to your hammers.... Here he is, Marvel's answer to John Henry ... The Mighty Thor!

Thor's Tried-and-True Back Kicks

(WE COULD HAVE CALLED THEM "KICKBACKS" BUT THOR WOULD NEVER HAVE ANYTHING TO DO WITH ANYTHING SHADY).

STANDING STRAIGHT, BEGIN TO LIFT EACH LEG AS IF YOU WERE MARCHING TO A COUNT OF TWELVE.

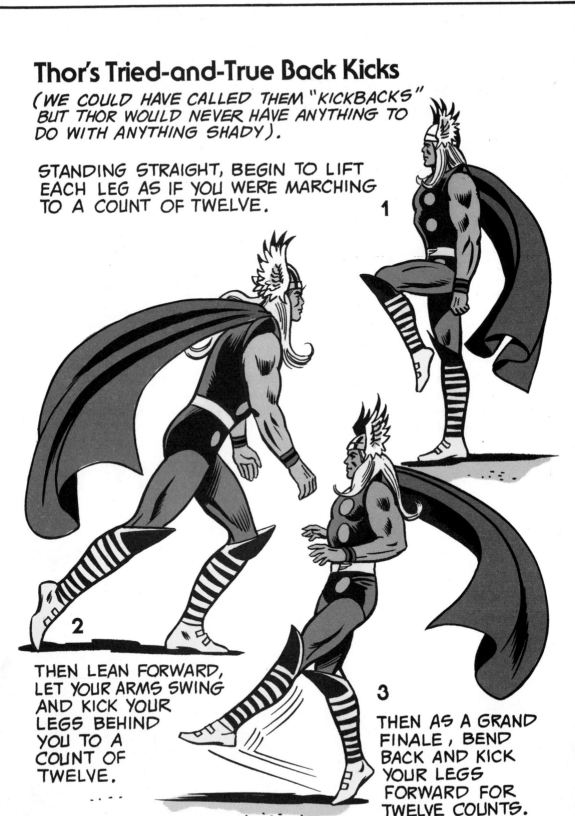

1

2

THEN LEAN FORWARD, LET YOUR ARMS SWING AND KICK YOUR LEGS BEHIND YOU TO A COUNT OF TWELVE.

3

THEN AS A GRAND FINALE, BEND BACK AND KICK YOUR LEGS FORWARD FOR TWELVE COUNTS.

Blondie's Just-So Rope Jumps

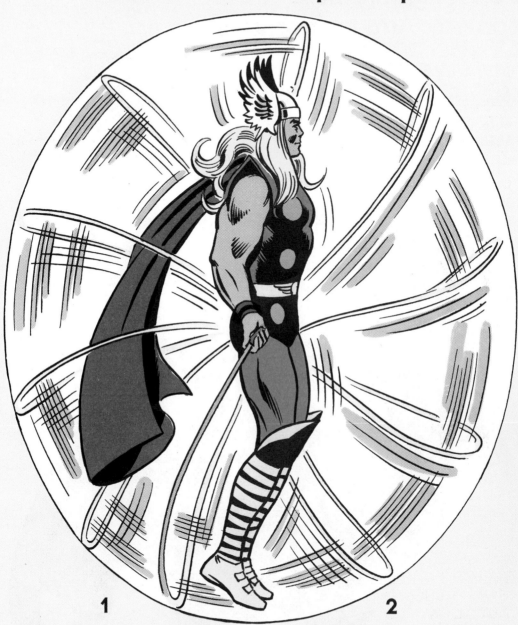

1

WE FIGURE YOU ALREADY
KNOW HOW TO JUMP ROPE,
SO NOW WE WANT YOU
TO USE ALL YOUR
EXPERTISE AND JUMP
20 TIMES, BOTH FEET
AT ONCE.

2

NOW, SLOW THE ROPE DOWN A
LITTLE AND TRY JUMPING
AN EXTRA TIME WHEN THE
ROPE IS OVERHEAD. WHEN
YOU HAVE THE RHYTHM OF
THIS, SPEED UP THE ROPE.
(THOR ALWAYS DID LIKE A
CHALLENGE).

Goldilocks' Greatest Isometric Arm Invigorators

IN A STANDING POSITION, CLASP YOUR HANDS TOGETHER NEAR YOUR CHEST WITH YOUR ELBOWS ON A STRAIGHT LINE WITH YOUR WRISTS.

1

PUSH YOUR HANDS TOGETHER WITH A MODERATE AMOUNT OF EXERTION AND HOLD FOR FIVE SECONDS. THEN INCREASE THE AMOUNT OF EXERTION AND THE LENGTH OF TIME GRADUALLY.

2

NOT EVEN HERCULES, SON OF ZEUS, CAN ABUSE HIS BODY WITH IMPUNITY.

3

THEN DO THE SAME THING, BUT LOCK YOUR HANDS BY CURVING YOUR FINGERS AND *PULL* THIS TIME INSTEAD OF PUSH!

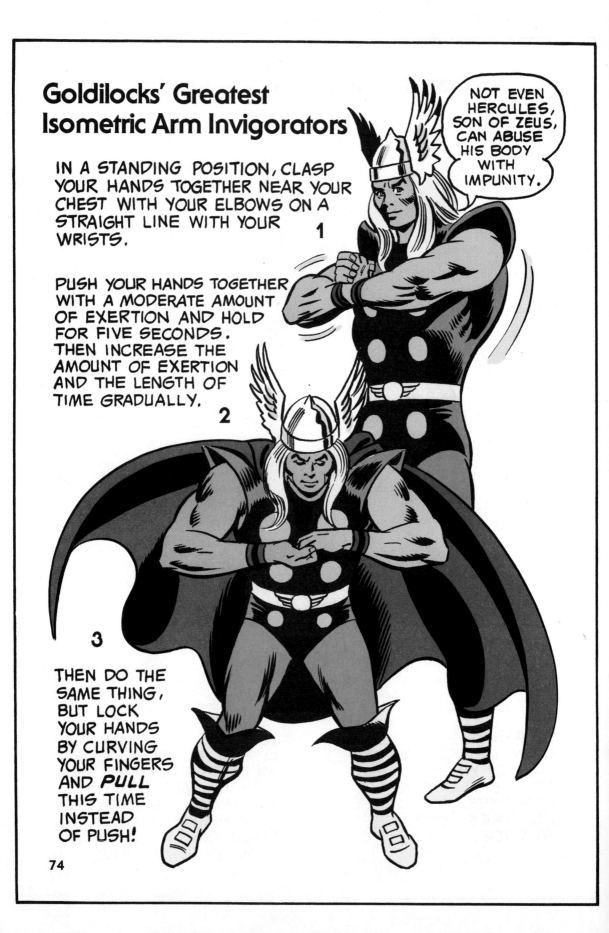

74

The Son of Odin Shoulder Strengthener

BEND YOUR LEFT ARM SO THAT YOUR FOREARM IS PARALLEL TO THE FLOOR. LOCK YOUR RIGHT AND LEFT HANDS SO THAT YOUR WRISTS ARE AT RIGHT ANGLES TO EACH OTHER.

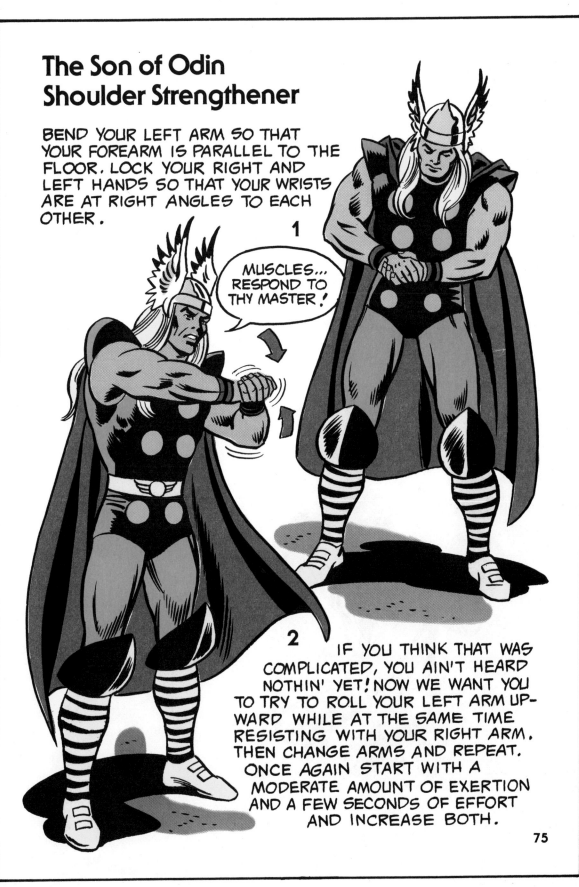

1

MUSCLES... RESPOND TO THY MASTER!

2

IF YOU THINK THAT WAS COMPLICATED, YOU AIN'T HEARD NOTHIN' YET! NOW WE WANT YOU TO TRY TO ROLL YOUR LEFT ARM UPWARD WHILE AT THE SAME TIME RESISTING WITH YOUR RIGHT ARM. THEN CHANGE ARMS AND REPEAT. ONCE AGAIN START WITH A MODERATE AMOUNT OF EXERTION AND A FEW SECONDS OF EFFORT AND INCREASE BOTH.

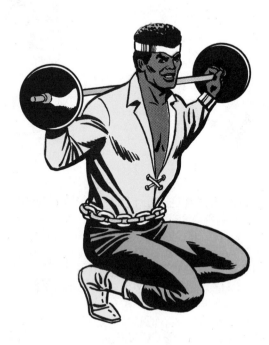

A LITTLE MUSCLE NEVER HURTS:

8

Power Plays from Power Man

This isn't the easiest chapter in the book, but then Power Man is tougher than most superheroes, reluctant or otherwise.

We wouldn't suggest that you ka-whump right into these exercises — not until you've been working on the others in the book for a month or so. Then start slowly and make sure you aren't hurting yourself by doing things your body isn't ready to do.

But once you tangle with ol' Lucas, you're apt to find yourself with strength beyond belief — and as the Hero himself might say . . . "That ain't half bad!"

Super Dude's Free Squats

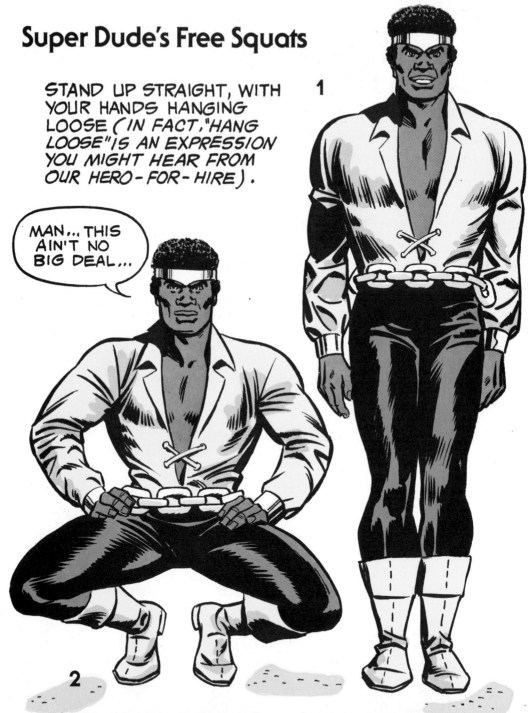

STAND UP STRAIGHT, WITH YOUR HANDS HANGING LOOSE (IN FACT, "HANG LOOSE" IS AN EXPRESSION YOU MIGHT HEAR FROM OUR HERO-FOR-HIRE).

1

MAN... THIS AIN'T NO BIG DEAL...

2

RAISE TO YOUR TOES AND SQUAT DOWN, KEEPING YOUR BACK AND HEAD PERFECTLY STRAIGHT. RETURN TO YOUR STARTING POSITION AND REPEAT.

Super Dude's Expensive Squats

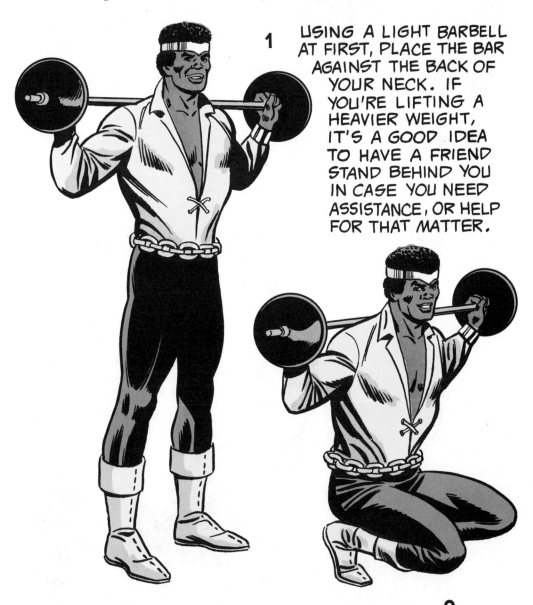

1 USING A LIGHT BARBELL AT FIRST, PLACE THE BAR AGAINST THE BACK OF YOUR NECK. IF YOU'RE LIFTING A HEAVIER WEIGHT, IT'S A GOOD IDEA TO HAVE A FRIEND STAND BEHIND YOU IN CASE YOU NEED ASSISTANCE, OR HELP FOR THAT MATTER.

2

NOW, IN ONE MOTION RAISE TO YOUR TOES AND SQUAT DOWN, KEEPING YOUR BACK AND HEAD PERFECTLY STRAIGHT. RETURN TO A STANDING POSITION AND REPEAT.

The Power Man Pull

1 USING LIGHT WEIGHTS AT FIRST, BEND AT THE WAIST KEEPING YOUR BACK PARALLEL TO THE GROUND AND YOUR LEGS AND BACK STRAIGHT.

2 IN ONE MOTION, PULL THE WEIGHT STRAIGHT UP TO NECK LEVEL, LETTING YOUR SHOULDERS AND ARMS DO ALL THE WORK.

3 GENTLY LOWER YOUR ARMS TO THEIR ORIGINAL POSITION. ONCE AGAIN, START WITH LIGHT WEIGHTS AND FEW REPETITIONS AND GRADUALLY WORK UP.

Cage's Calf Crusher

STAND UP STRAIGHT, YOUR FEET COMFORTABLY APART.
HOLD THE BARBELL NEXT TO THE INSIDE CORNERS
AND REST THE BAR ACROSS YOUR SHOULDERS.

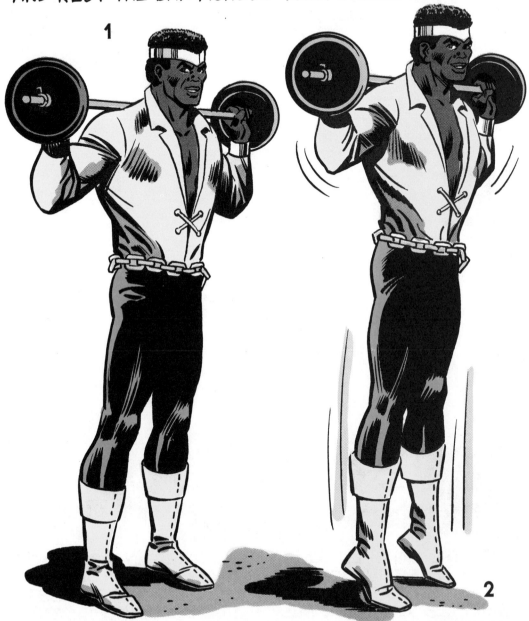

SLOWLY RAISE TO YOUR TOES KEEPING YOUR LEGS
AND BACK STRAIGHT. START WITH A DOZEN AND WORK UP.

Luke's Lying-Down Limb Lifter

LIE ON YOUR BACK, CROSS YOUR ANKLES (BUT DON'T HOPE TO DIE) AND BRING YOUR KNEES UP TO YOUR CHEST. HOLD A LIGHT BARBELL ON THE FLOOR BEHIND YOUR HEAD.

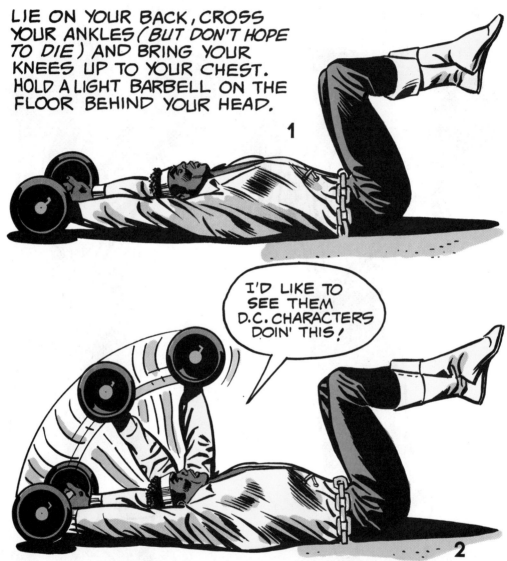

I'D LIKE TO SEE THEM D.C. CHARACTERS DOIN' THIS!

LIFT THE BARBELL TO A POINT DIRECTLY ABOVE YOUR CHEST, KEEPING YOUR ARMS AND BACK STRAIGHT AND YOUR FEET OFF THE FLOOR. YOUR SIDE AND CHEST MUSCLES ARE THE ONES YOU'LL BE USING IF YOU DO THE EXERCISE CORRECTLY--OR EVEN IF YOU JUST DO IT RIGHT. RETURN TO YOUR STARTING POSITION AND REPEAT.

The "You talking to me?" Shrug

(FOR USE BY PEOPLE
WHEN CONFRONTED BY
AUTHORITY FIGURES)

1 STAND UP STRAIGHT (SHEESH!
ARE WE SICK OF WRITING
THAT ONE!) FEET COMFORT-
ABLY APART. (THAT, TOO)
HOLD THE WEIGHTS IN YOUR
HANDS, BY YOUR THIGHS.

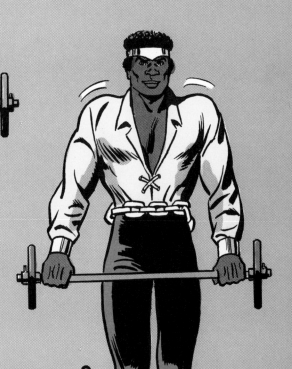

KEEPING YOUR ARMS STRAIGHT,
RAISE YOUR SHOULDERS UP
SLOWLY AS IF YOU WERE
SHRUGGING OFF A QUESTION
YOU DIDN'T KNOW THE ANSWER
TO. START WITH LIGHT WEIGHTS
AND WORK UP TO HEAVIER
WEIGHTS AND MORE REPETITIONS.

2

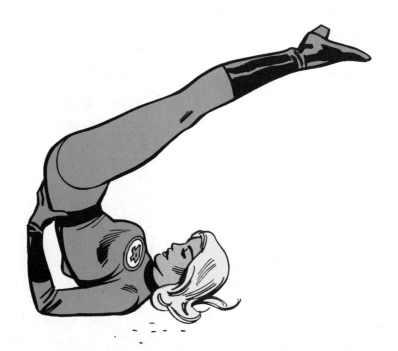

YOU'RE A SHADOW OF YOUR FORMER SELF:

9

A Slimming Program from The Invisible Girl

You'd think with her busy schedule, Sue Storm would never have time to eat, much less gain weight. But even the most fantastic of us occasionally has to fight off a few extra pounds, and Sue is all too eager to share her secrets of weight control with us.

So put down that Big Mac and turn the page. If Dr. Atkins can do it, so can Marvel!

What's a Nice Girl Like You Doing in a Weight Class Like This? (a Discussion of What Puts On Weight)

We hate to be killjoys, or even killravens, but in almost every case, fat people or even slightly fat people are that way because they eat more food than their activity requires.

Food is fuel, just like the gas you put in your car. If you drive a lot, you'll be putting in more and more gasoline (unless there's an energy crisis, in which case this whole explanation bites the dust). If you keep putting gas in your car, even though you're not driving it, the gas will overflow onto the ground, making the ground very wet and smelly and making your Sunoco dealer very unfriendly.

If you keep eating, even though you're not moving around, the extra food you eat will have no place to go, and instead of spilling onto your Sunoco dealer's driveway, it spills over onto your waistline and becomes fat.

So the way to maintain your weight is to eat the same amount of food that your body needs to keep you moving around. If you want to lose weight, you have to either eat less or move around more or a little of both.

The energy food contains is measured in a little thing called a calorie. If something is said to contain 50 calories, it will give your body twice as much energy to burn as something containing 25 calories.

But there's one catch. Some foods do terrific things for your body and some foods do nothing good for you, and some dumb kids think the good foods don't taste as good as the no-good foods. (Good foods often hang out in the fruit, dairy, vegetable and meat sections of your supermarkets, and bad foods are often found at the candy counters and in the movie theaters.)

There's probably nothing wrong with an occasional Three Musketeers (we're slightly partial to them ourselves), but you should concentrate on fueling your body with the best foods possible, the foods with the most nutritional value — which often happen, O Lucky Person, to be the foods with the least calories.

But there's one warning: every calorie you take in has to be burned up to keep you from gaining weight, and it doesn't matter if that calorie came along in a milkshake or a beansprout. For every candy bar you eat, doing your body almost no good but contributing about 200 calories, you could eat a hamburger and a salad, doing great things for your body and giving you the exact same number of calories to use up.

So any mature, self-controlled, perfect person knows it makes sense to stick to the good foods (fruits, vegetables, meats, fish, poultry and dairy products) and lay off the sweets . . . except on birthdays, bar mitzvahs, trips to Disneyland and other special occasions.

The following pages will give you an idea of what foods have how many calories. Remember that the calorie values listed are just for the foods listed. A hot dog is only 125 calories, but if you add a roll and ketchup, you've added 200 calores more. So, as the lithe Ms. Storm would say, don't fool yourself . . . because there's no foolin' the bathroom scale.

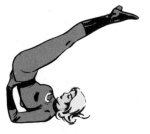 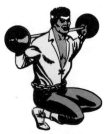 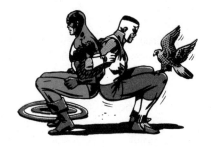 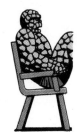

Sue's Colossal

Almonds (each)	10
American cheese (one slice)	75
Animal crackers (six, including the hippo)	50
Apple (medium)	60
Apple juice (small glass)	60
Apple pie (one slice)	350
Applesauce (1/2 cup)	90
Apricots, canned (three halves)	60
Bacon (two slices)	100
Bacon, lettuce and tomato sandwich	300
Baked beans (one cup)	200
Banana	130
Beans, green (one cup)	50
Beef stew (one cup)	250
Beer	Are you kidding?
Bologna (one slice)	65
Bran, raisin (one cup)	150
Bread (one slice)	75
Broccoli (one cup)	45
Brownie (one medium)	140
Butter (one pat)	70
Butterscotch candy (one)	20
Cake (one piece angel food)	120
Cake (one piece layer)	350
Cantaloupe (1/2)	30
Caramel (one)	45
Carrot (one)	20
Celery (one stalk)	10
Cherries (20 fresh)	60
Cherry pie (one slice)	360
Chewing gum (one stick)	8
Chicken, broiled or roasted (1/2 small)	100
Chicken, fried (1/2 small)	275
Chicken noodle soup (one cup)	125
Chili (1/2 cup)	150
Chocolate bar (one ounce)	155
Chocolate cookie (most large)	75
Chocolate cupcake (one, with icing)	250
Chocolate milkshake	420

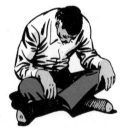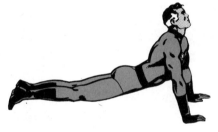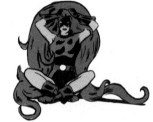

Calorie Counter

Cinnamon bun	170
Cola (eight ounces)	100
Coleslaw (one cup)	150
Corn (one ear)	90
Cornflakes (one bowl)	110
Cottage cheese (1/2 cup)	175
Cucumber (one)	15
Doughnut (one)	200
Egg, boiled (one average)	75
Egg, fried or scrambled (one average)	125
Flounder, fried (average serving)	200
Frankfurter	125
French bread (1-inch slice)	55
Fruit cocktail (six tablespoons w/juice)	70
Gelatin dessert	75
Graham crackers (three)	110
Grapefruit (1/2)	75
Grapes (one cup)	100
Gravy (one tablespoon)	40
Ham (average serving)	250
Hamburger (small, no bun)	150
Honey (one tablespoon)	60
Hot dog (a frankfurter by any other name)	125
Ice cream (average scoop)	150
Ice cream sundae (average, goopy)	400
Jams and jellies (one tablespoon)	50
Ketchup (one tablespoon)	15
Lamb chop (two small)	250
Lemon (one medium)	20
Lemon meringue pie (one slice)	350
Lettuce (two or three leaves)	5

(No wonder you've never seen a fat rabbit!)

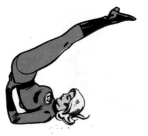 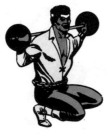 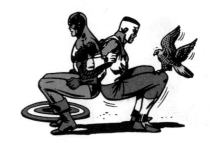 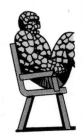

Sue's Colossal

Life Saver (one)	10
Limburger cheese	Yuk!
Liver (enough to keep your mom quiet)	85
Lobster (one average)	300
Macaroni (one cup, cooked)	155
Maple syrup (one tablespoon, dripped)	50
Marshmallow (one)	25
Mayonnaise (one tablespoon)	60
Meat loaf (one large slice)	265
Milk, whole (eight ounces)	165
Milk, skimmed (eight ounces)	85
Muffin, English	150
Mustard (one tablespoon)	10
Nectarines (two average)	60
Noodles (one cup, cooked)	150
Nuts, mixed (eight to twelve)	95
Oil, salad (one tablespoon)	125
Olives, green (one)	8
Olives, ripe (one)	10
Onion (small, raw ... whew!)	50
Orange (one medium)	75
Orange juice (small glass)	65
Peach (one medium)	35
Peach, canned in syrup	80
Pear (one medium)	70
Pear, canned in syrup	95
Peanut butter (one tablespoon)	90
Peanut butter and jelly sandwich	290
Peanuts (16 fresh roasted)	85
Peanuts, canned and salted (1/2 cup)	670
Peas (1/2 cup)	55
Pickle, dill (one large)	15
Pickle, sweet (one small)	20
Pigeon	Who could eat a pigeon?
Pineapple (one slice, canned in syrup)	80
Plum, red (one)	30

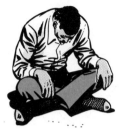 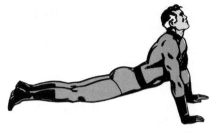 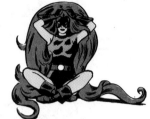

Calorie Counter

Pork chop (one)	200
Potato, baked (one)	100
Potatoes, French-fried (1/2 cup)	310
Potato chip (one ... but nobody can eat just one)	10
Pretzel (one medium)	70
Puffed cereals (one cup, no sugar)	50
Radish (one)	2
Raisins (1/2 cup)	300
Rice (1/2 cup, cooked)	100
Roast beef sandwich (cold)	340
Salami (one large slice)	130
Sandwich (average ... now, what's so average about a sandwich?)	350
Sausage (one 3-inch link)	95
Shrimp, fresh (one)	10
Spinach (1/2 cup)	25
Squash, yellow (1/2 cup)	15
Strawberries (one fresh)	4
Strawberries, frozen (1/2 cup)	90
Strawberry shortcake	400
Sugar (one tablespoon)	50
Sweet potato, baked (one)	185
Sweet potato, candied (one)	350
Swiss cheese (one slice)	65
Tangerine (one large)	45
Tomato (one medium)	30
Tomato soup (big bowl)	110
Tuna salad sandwich	340
Turkey (two slices)	185
Vanilla wafer	20
Veal cutlet, breaded (one medium)	215
Vegetable soup (big bowl)	100
Waffle (one)	220
Watermelon (one slice)	20
Yoghurt, plain (one cup)	130

Sue's Super Seat Slimmers

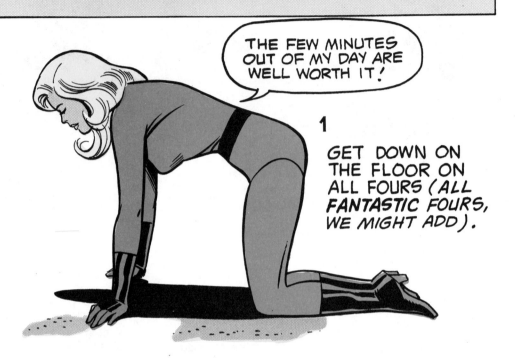

THE FEW MINUTES OUT OF MY DAY ARE WELL WORTH IT!

1 GET DOWN ON THE FLOOR ON ALL FOURS (*ALL FANTASTIC FOURS*, WE MIGHT ADD).

2 SLOWLY RAISE YOUR LEFT LEG AS HIGH AS YOU CAN AND HOLD TO A COUNT OF SIX.

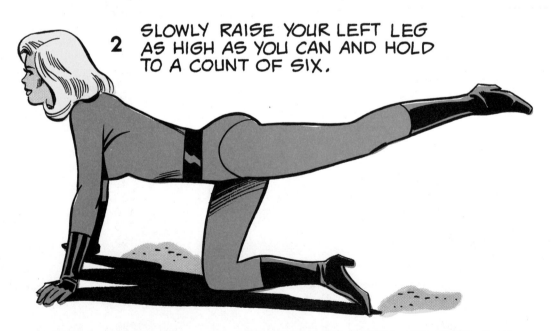

LOWER YOUR LEFT LEG AND REPEAT WITH YOUR RIGHT.

The Fantastic One-Two-Three-Four

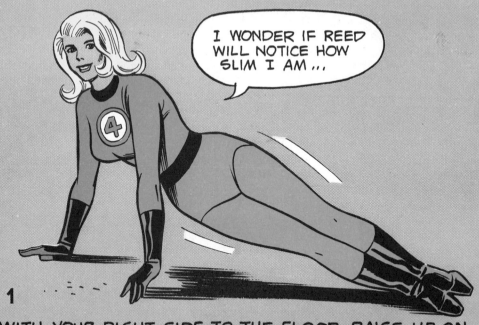

1

WITH YOUR RIGHT SIDE TO THE FLOOR, RAISE UP ON RIGHT ARM AND THE SIDE OF YOUR RIGHT FOOT, BALANCING WITH YOUR LEFT ARM IF YOU NEED TO.

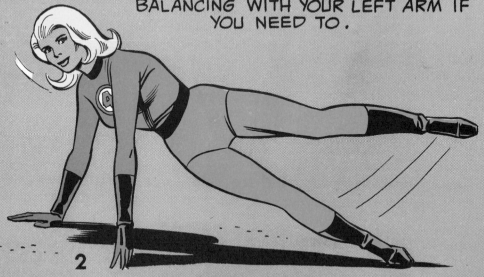

2

RAISE YOUR LEFT LEG UP UNTIL IT'S PARALLEL WITH THE FLOOR, HOLD FOR A COUNT OF ONE-TWO-THREE-FOUR (*NOW DO YOU SEE HOW THE EXERCISE GOT ITS NAME*) AND RETURN TO YOUR STARTING POSITION. REPEAT SEVERAL TIMES, AND THEN FLIP OVER AND DO THE SAME EXERCISE ON YOUR LEFT SIDE.

Storm's Savage Stomach Sizer

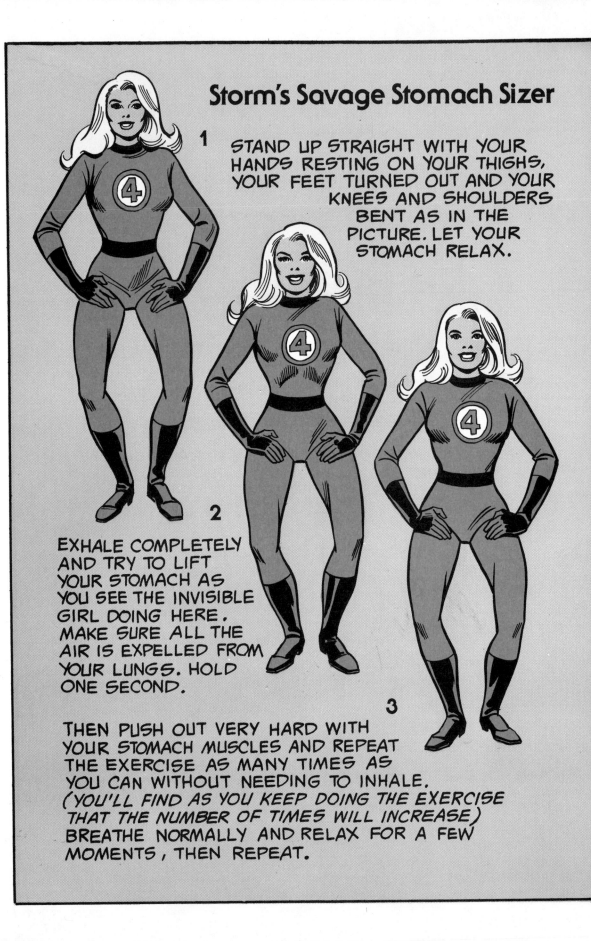

1 STAND UP STRAIGHT WITH YOUR HANDS RESTING ON YOUR THIGHS, YOUR FEET TURNED OUT AND YOUR KNEES AND SHOULDERS BENT AS IN THE PICTURE. LET YOUR STOMACH RELAX.

2 EXHALE COMPLETELY AND TRY TO LIFT YOUR STOMACH AS YOU SEE THE INVISIBLE GIRL DOING HERE. MAKE SURE ALL THE AIR IS EXPELLED FROM YOUR LUNGS. HOLD ONE SECOND.

3 THEN PUSH OUT VERY HARD WITH YOUR STOMACH MUSCLES AND REPEAT THE EXERCISE AS MANY TIMES AS YOU CAN WITHOUT NEEDING TO INHALE. (YOU'LL FIND AS YOU KEEP DOING THE EXERCISE THAT THE NUMBER OF TIMES WILL INCREASE) BREATHE NORMALLY AND RELAX FOR A FEW MOMENTS, THEN REPEAT.

The Sue Storm Shoulder Stand

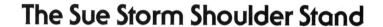

1 LIE ON YOUR BACK WITH YOUR HANDS AT YOUR SIDES AND YOUR BODY RELAXED.

2 PLACE YOUR PALMS HARD AGAINST THE FLOOR, AND USING YOUR LEG AND STOMACH MUSCLES, SLOWLY RAISE YOUR LEGS OFF THE FLOOR.

3 USING YOUR HANDS TO PROP UP YOUR HIPS, SWING YOUR LEGS BACK SO YOUR HIPS LEAVE THE FLOOR.

SLOWLY STRAIGHTEN UP AND WHEN YOU FEEL YOU CAN'T COMFORTABLY GO ANY FURTHER, HOLD YOUR POSITION FOR SEVERAL MINUTES. YOUR EYES SHOULD BE CLOSED AND YOUR BODY RELAXED. 4

TO COME OUT OF THE SHOULDER STAND, DON'T JUST DROP TO THE FLOOR. BEND YOUR KNEES, PUT YOUR HANDS BACK ON THE FLOOR AND ROLL FORWARD SLOWLY, ARCHING YOUR NECK BACK— WARD SO YOUR HEAD STAYS ON THE FLOOR. WHEN YOUR BACK IS FLAT ON THE FLOOR AND YOUR LEGS STRAIGHT UP, VERY SLOWLY LOWER YOUR LEGS TO THE FLOOR. THEN RELAX COMPLETELY. THIS EXERCISE SHOULD ONLY BE DONE ONCE A DAY.

5

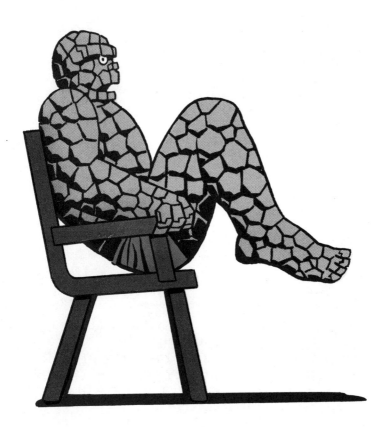

IT'S FAT-CLOBBERING TIME:

10

Thing's Tried-and-True Tirade Against Unsightly Lumps and Bumps

Well, nobody knows better than Ben Grimm how grim a fellow (or a girl fellow) can feel when bumps and lumps obscure an otherwise perfect physique (we've been grim about that situation a few times ourselves, we add ever so cleverly).

Even if your lumps and bumps aren't bright orange, you'd probably gladly trade your FOOM subscription for a sleek smooth body to match your sleek smooth personality.

But we wouldn't make you go to those extremes, would we ...? Aw, c'mon ... would we? Nope. Of course not, and why would you even ask such a question?

What we _are_ going to do is allow your old friend Ben, affectionately known as The Thing, to teach you how to tackle those unsightly bulges like he tackles the arch enemies who plague him and his cavorting cronies.

So for these and other marvelous answers to questions of fat and slim, we proudly present Chapter Ten.

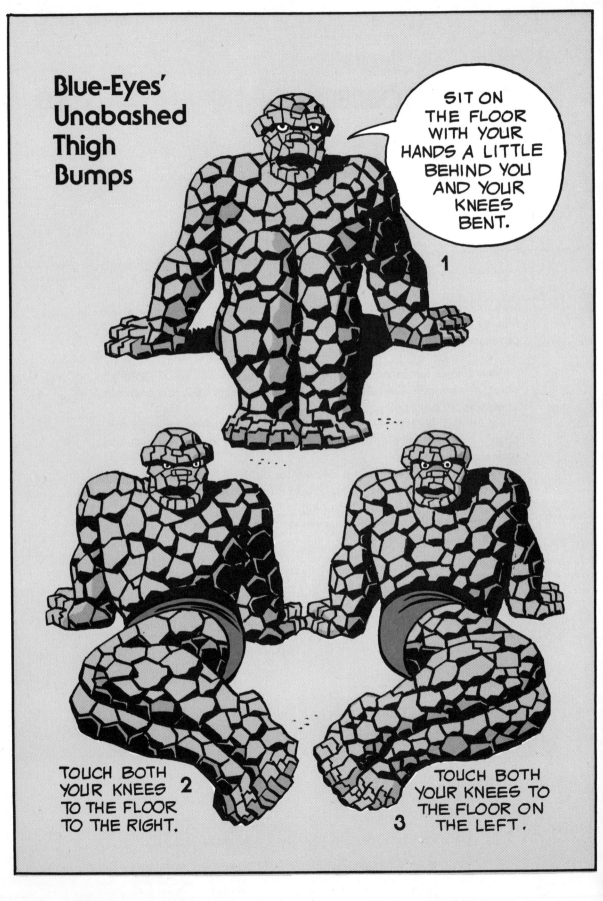

Thing's Thoroughbred Thigh Thinner

SIT ON THE FLOOR WITH YOUR KNEES UP AND YOUR HANDS SLIGHTLY BEHIND YOU (IF THIS SOUNDS FAMILIAR, IT'S BECAUSE YOU JUST DID IT IN THE LAST EXERCISE).

1

2 ROLL TO YOUR RIGHT SIDE BUT DON'T LET YOUR KNEES TOUCH THE FLOOR.

I'D LIKE TO MEET THE GUY WHO THOUGHT THIS ONE UP!

STRETCH OUT YOUR LEGS IN FRONT OF YOU. **3**

4

HOLD FOR A SECOND, BEND YOUR KNEES AND REPEAT ON YOUR LEFT SIDE.

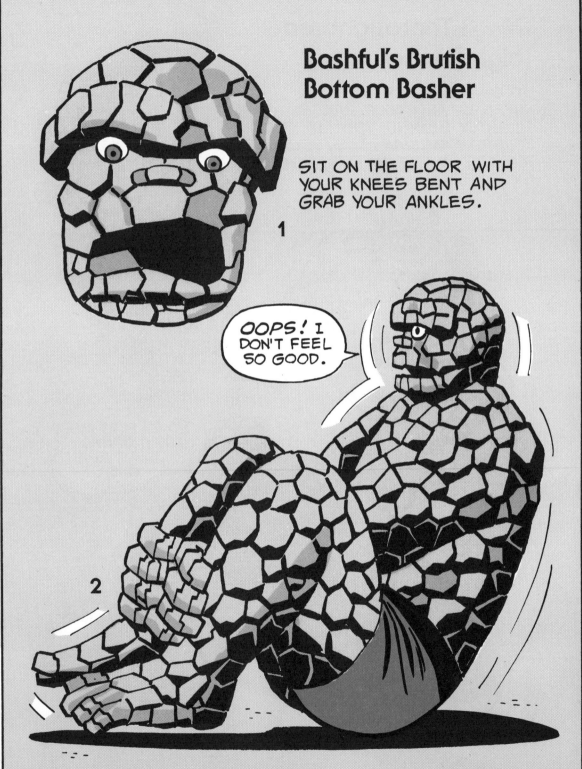

Bashful's Brutish Bottom Basher

SIT ON THE FLOOR WITH YOUR KNEES BENT AND GRAB YOUR ANKLES.

1

OOPS! I DON'T FEEL SO GOOD.

2

ROCK BACK AND FORTH, UNTIL YOU START TO FEEL SEASICK.

Orange Skin's Sedentary Stomach Squelcher

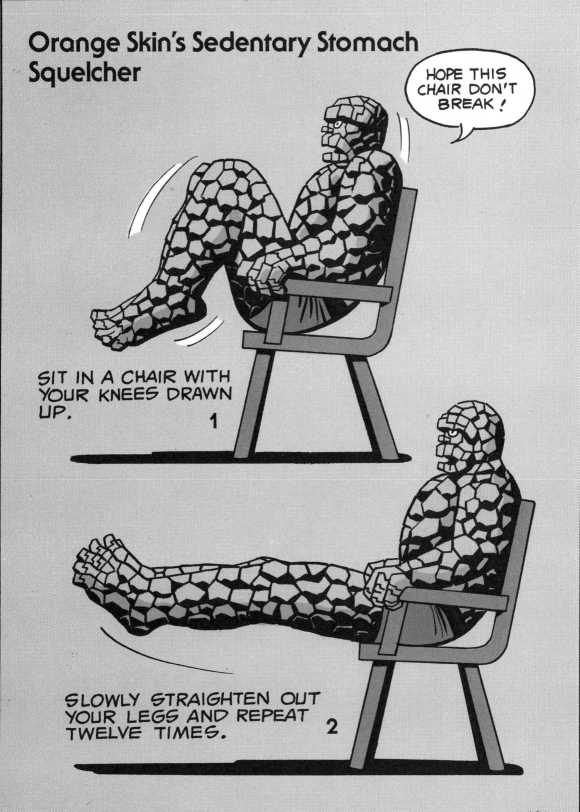

SIT IN A CHAIR WITH YOUR KNEES DRAWN UP.
1

SLOWLY STRAIGHTEN OUT YOUR LEGS AND REPEAT TWELVE TIMES.
2

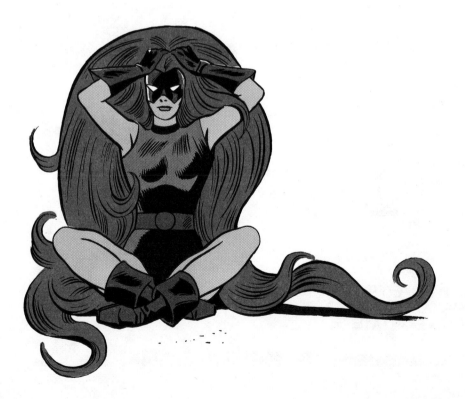

I'LL HAVE TO SAY I LOVE YOU IN A SAUNA:

11

Beauty and Health-Care Tips from
Medusa (Marvel's answer to
Lauren Hutton)

As far as we're concerned, when it comes to beauty, no one can hold a candle to Medusa. No mere 100 strokes a night could make hair that super, and you just don't find skin that clear on your everyday, run-of-the-mill android.

We can't promise you hair and skin like Medusa's, but we can give you a few of her secrets, and with a little extra help from Mr. Revlon, how can you go wrong?

Medusa's Magnificent Mandible Movers

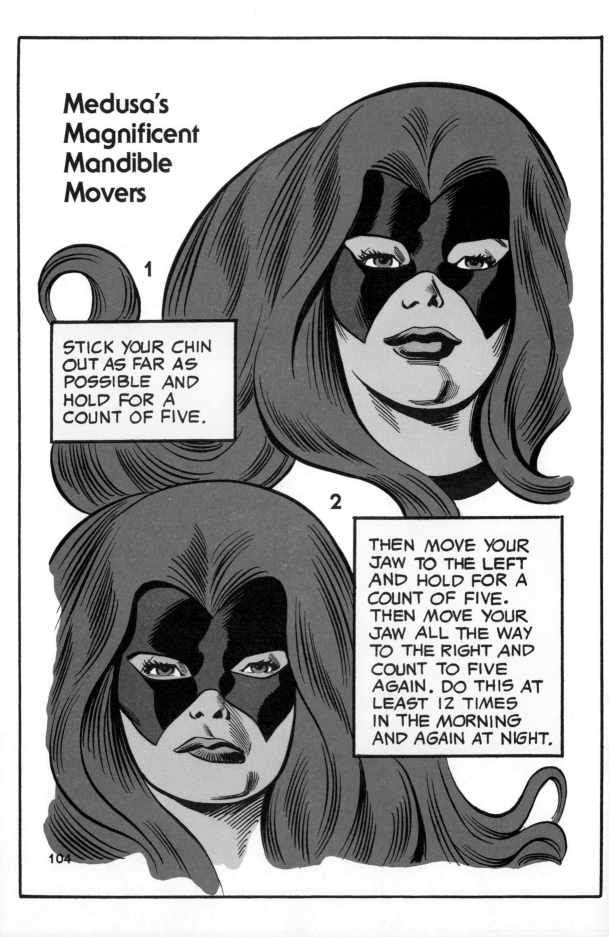

1

STICK YOUR CHIN OUT AS FAR AS POSSIBLE AND HOLD FOR A COUNT OF FIVE.

2

THEN MOVE YOUR JAW TO THE LEFT AND HOLD FOR A COUNT OF FIVE. THEN MOVE YOUR JAW ALL THE WAY TO THE RIGHT AND COUNT TO FIVE AGAIN. DO THIS AT LEAST 12 TIMES IN THE MORNING AND AGAIN AT NIGHT.

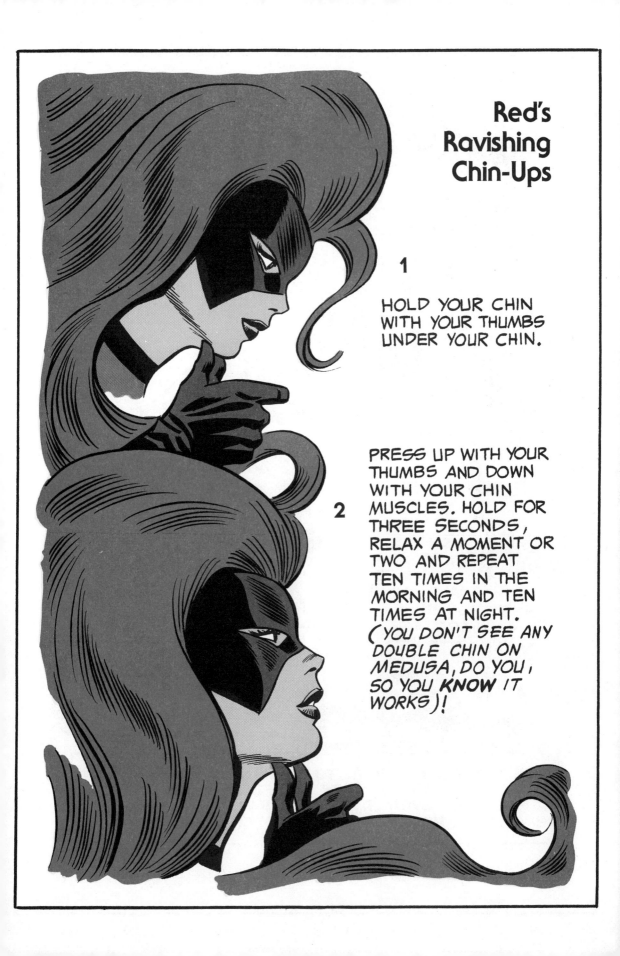

Red's Ravishing Chin-Ups

1

HOLD YOUR CHIN WITH YOUR THUMBS UNDER YOUR CHIN.

2

PRESS UP WITH YOUR THUMBS AND DOWN WITH YOUR CHIN MUSCLES. HOLD FOR THREE SECONDS, RELAX A MOMENT OR TWO AND REPEAT TEN TIMES IN THE MORNING AND TEN TIMES AT NIGHT. *(YOU DON'T SEE ANY DOUBLE CHIN ON MEDUSA, DO YOU, SO YOU **KNOW** IT WORKS)!*

Fiery's Furious Follicle Flourisher

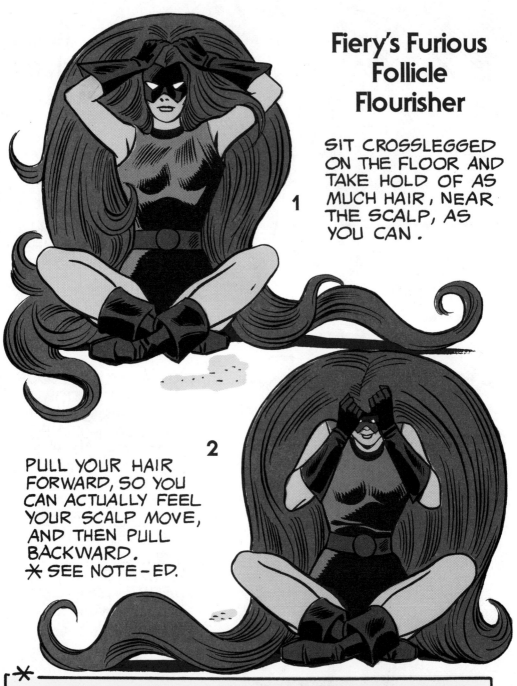

1 SIT CROSSLEGGED ON THE FLOOR AND TAKE HOLD OF AS MUCH HAIR, NEAR THE SCALP, AS YOU CAN.

2 PULL YOUR HAIR FORWARD, SO YOU CAN ACTUALLY FEEL YOUR SCALP MOVE, AND THEN PULL BACKWARD.
✳ SEE NOTE – ED.

✳
DON'T TRY TO DO THIS TO A FRIEND OR TEACHER WITHOUT GETTING HIS OR HER PERMISSION FIRST. A FOE WILL NEVER GIVE YOU PERMISSION IF HE HAS BRAINS, OR HAIR FOR THAT MATTER – ED.

The "I Only Have Eyes for You"

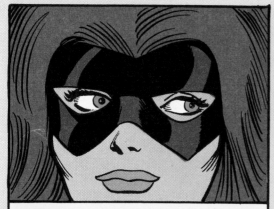

OPEN YOUR EYES VERY WIDE AND ROLL YOUR EYES AS FAR AS YOU CAN TO THE LEFT. HOLD ONE SECOND.

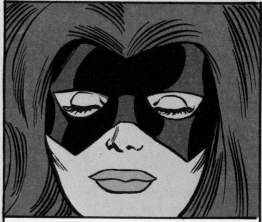

THEN ROLL YOUR EYES TO THE BOTTOM AND HOLD ONE SECOND.

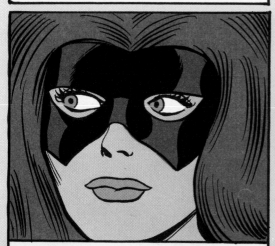

THEN TO THE RIGHT AND HOLD ONE SECOND.

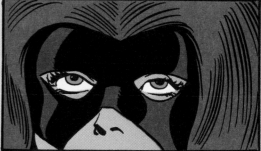

AND FINALLY ROLL THOSE BABY BLUES, IF YOU *HAVE* BABY BLUES *(SEE NOTE)* TO THE TOP AND HOLD ONE SECOND. DO THIS TEN TIMES CLOCKWISE AND TEN TIMES COUNTER CLOCKWISE.

NOTE: THE DECISION ON WHETHER TO ALLOW PEOPLE *(OR SUPERHEROES)* WITH BROWN, GREEN OR HAZEL EYES *(OR ONE OF EACH)* TO DO THIS EXERCISE IS STILL PENDING IN THE GREAT REFUGE SUPREME COURT. AS THE HULK WOULD NEVER THINK OF SAYING "*THE WHEELS OF JUSTICE GRIND EXCEEDINGLY SLOW.*"

The Second-Greatest Refuge

(MEDUSA'S MAGICAL ANGLE BOARD AND HOW TO MAKE ONE)

AS EVERYONE FROM CLEOPATRA (WHO *IS* THIS CLEOPATRA...? SHE MUST BE A D.C. CHARACTER) TO RED SONYA KNOWS, YOU'VE *GOT* TO HAVE AN ANGLE! SO HERE'S MEDUSA'S NEW SLANT ON LIFE, A BOARD SHE BUILT HERSELF (WITH ALL DUE RESPECT, SHE *DID* BORROW THOR'S HAMMER AND SOME NAILS FROM IRON MAN).

AN ANGLE BOARD ONLY WORKS IF YOU LIE DOWN ON IT FROM TIME TO TIME, PREFERABLY FOR TEN OR FIFTEEN MINUTES. (IN OTHER WORDS, IT DOESN'T DO *ANYTHING* FOR YOU IF YOU LEAVE IT IN YOUR CLOSET.) AT THE END OF THE DAY, IT'LL HELP YOU RELAX, AND ANY TIME IT'LL WORK MAGIC FOR YOUR COMPLEXION AND HAIR BY INCREASING THE AMOUNT OF BLOOD REACHING YOUR HEAD.

HERE ARE SOME RATHER HAP-HAZZARD INSTRUCTIONS ON MAKING AN ANGLE BOARD OF YOUR OWN. SO MAKE ONE TODAY, AND DO A GOOD TURN FOR THE LUMBER INDUSTRY (AND ALSO FOR YOURSELF).

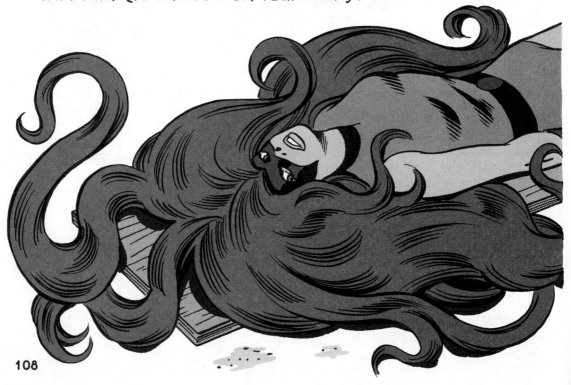

MATERIALS

BOARD 3/4" INTERIOR PLYWOOD 6' LONG X 1½' WIDE
LEGS AND BRACES 2 X 4 8' LONG
NAILS OR WOOD SCREWS
SANDPAPER

DIRECTIONS

PROP BOARD END TO ABOUT 16" HIGH. POSITION LEGS
NEXT TO BOARD AS ILLUSTRATED. MARK ANGLE TO BE
CUT, AND USE THIS ANGLE AS A TEMPLET FOR THE
OTHER LEG.

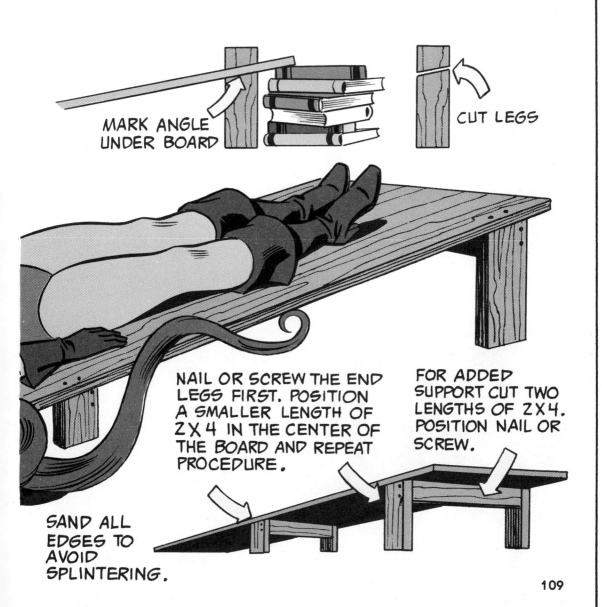

MARK ANGLE
UNDER BOARD

CUT LEGS

NAIL OR SCREW THE END
LEGS FIRST. POSITION
A SMALLER LENGTH OF
2 X 4 IN THE CENTER OF
THE BOARD AND REPEAT
PROCEDURE.

FOR ADDED
SUPPORT CUT TWO
LENGTHS OF 2 X 4.
POSITION NAIL OR
SCREW.

SAND ALL
EDGES TO
AVOID
SPLINTERING.

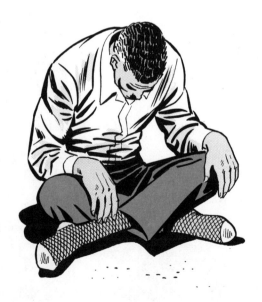

HOW TO UNWIND, 12
FORGIVE AND
FORGET:
Relaxation Exercises from
J. Jonah Jameson

Now, anybody who's perused a few issues of The Amazing Spider-Man can attest to the fact that J. Jonah Jameson does not possess your typical low-key FM personality.

But we have inside information that J. Jonah's been slipping out to the health club once or twice a week in a desperate attempt to get his head together and relax between tantrums.

We're not claiming that things are easy for our parsimonious publisher. In comparison with Perry White's gig at the Planet, being publisher of the Daily Bugle is like being sentenced to a decade of Sunday mornings with Bob McAllister. In fact, we should send Bob a copy of this book.

But we don't know anybody who doesn't have a worry or two. Why, even Margaux Hemingway must get a pimple every now and then. So, Margaux, if you want to learn how to get your mind off your problems and how to unwind after a day as a superstar, just lend an ear.

El Cheapo's Back and Neck Rest

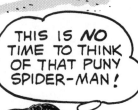

1 SIT INDIAN STYLE ON THE FLOOR, GRABBING YOUR TOES WITH YOUR HANDS.

DROP YOUR HEAD BACK FOR A COUNT OF SIX, TRYING TO RELAX THE MUSCLES OF YOUR NECK AND BACK.

2

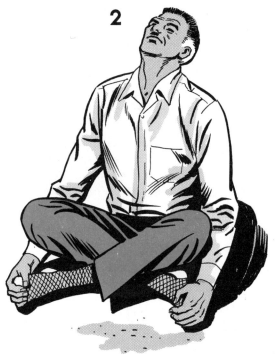

THIS IS *NO* TIME TO THINK OF THAT PUNY SPIDER-MAN!

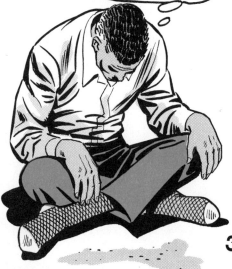

LET YOUR HEAD FALL FORWARD AND REST YOUR HANDS ON YOUR KNEES FOR A COUNT OF TEN.

3

The Jameson Roar

KNEEL ON THE FLOOR WITH YOUR BOTTOM RESTING ON YOUR HEELS AND YOUR HANDS ON YOUR THIGHS, PALMS DOWN.

1

BEND FORWARD, OPEN YOUR EYES AS WIDE AS YOU CAN, AND TENSE UP EVERY MUSCLE IN YOUR BODY.

2

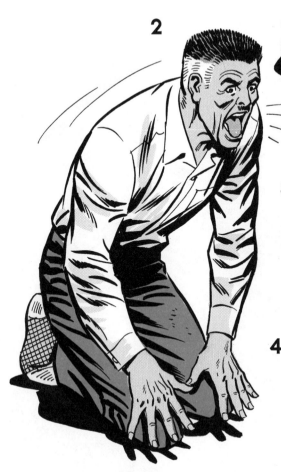

3 STICK YOUR TONGUE OUT AS FAR AS YOU CAN, SPREAD YOUR FINGERS WIDE APART AND HOLD TENSE FOR A COUNT OF 12.

4 SLOWLY RELAX, BRING YOUR TONGUE BACK WHERE IT BELONGS AND RETURN TO YOUR STARTING POSITION.

113

The Final Results of the Daily Bugle's "How I Get the Kinks Out" Contest

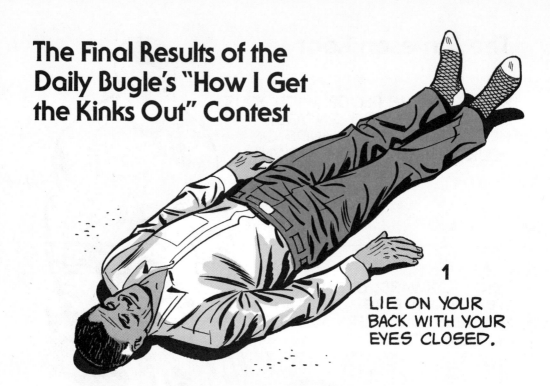

1

LIE ON YOUR BACK WITH YOUR EYES CLOSED.

STARTING AT YOUR FEET SYSTEMATICALLY RELAX EVERY MUSCLE UNTIL YOU REACH YOUR HEAD.

2

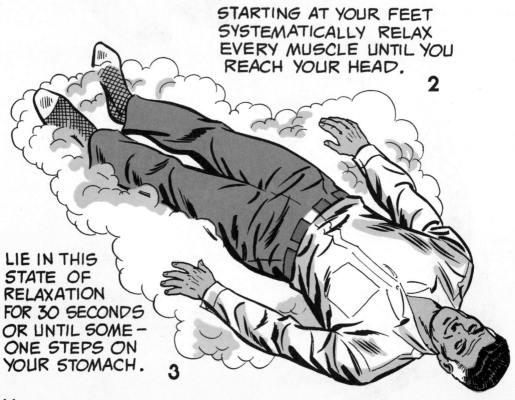

LIE IN THIS STATE OF RELAXATION FOR 30 SECONDS OR UNTIL SOME-ONE STEPS ON YOUR STOMACH.

3

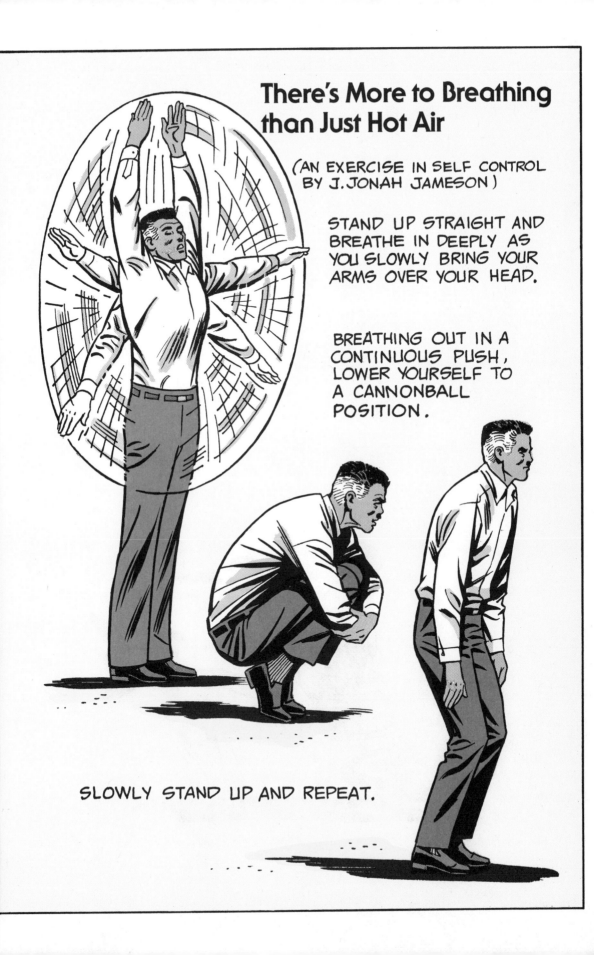

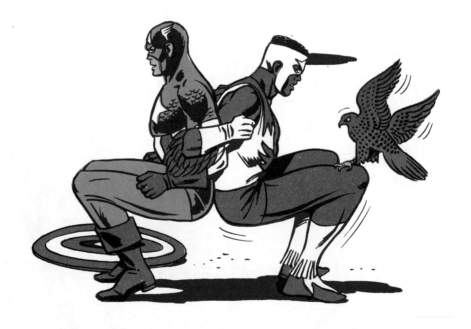

TWO CAN EXERCISE AS CHEAPLY AS ONE:

13

A Venture into Healthful Togetherness with Marvel's Musclebound Madcaps, Captain America and Falcon

Nothing like a little togetherness to cure the Bicentennial red-white-and-blues, or any other form of the blues you might be singing or feeling.

So here come those pertinacious proponents of patriotism themselves, Cap and Falcon, to show you a few exercises you can do with a friend — since the way we figure it, you spend too much time by yourself reading comic books anyway.

If you don't have a sidekick, go round one up and help each other get healthier and happier by doing the exercises on the next few pages.

The All-American Give and Take

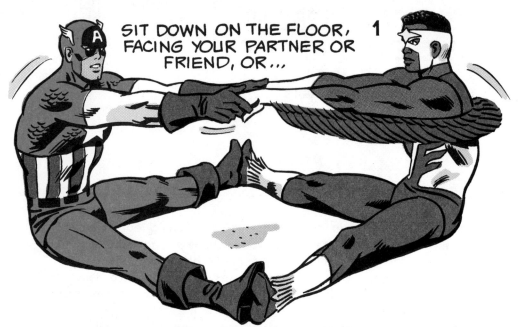

SIT DOWN ON THE FLOOR, 1
FACING YOUR PARTNER OR
FRIEND, OR...

BROTHER, OR ANYONE YOU MIGHT HAVE HANDY. JOIN
HANDS AND SPREAD YOUR LEGS WIDE APART, SO
THAT YOUR FEET ARE TOUCHING YOUR PARTNER'S
FEET.

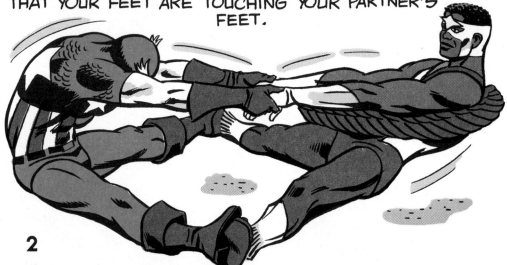

2

NOW ONE OF YOU SHOULD BEGIN TO LEAN BACK
SLOWLY, PULLING THE OTHER AS HE LEANS. THEN
THE OTHER ONE OF YOU SHOULD RECIPROCATE OR
IF HE'D PREFER, HE SHOULD RETURN THE FAVOR.
DO THIS FOR A DOZEN OR SO TIMES OR UNTIL YOUR
PARTNER STARTS MAKING INSULTING REMARKS.

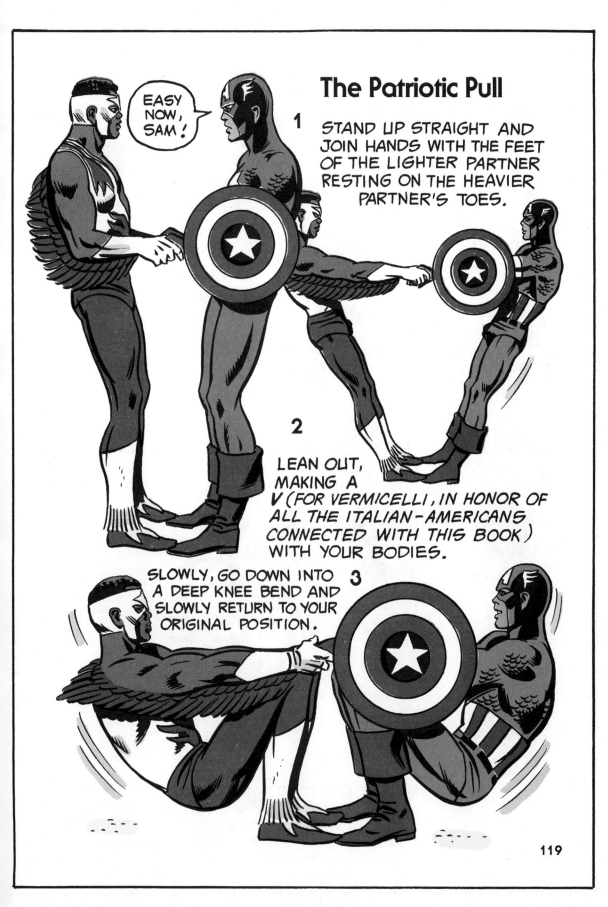

The Patriotic Pull

1 STAND UP STRAIGHT AND JOIN HANDS WITH THE FEET OF THE LIGHTER PARTNER RESTING ON THE HEAVIER PARTNER'S TOES.

2 LEAN OUT, MAKING A V (FOR VERMICELLI, IN HONOR OF ALL THE ITALIAN-AMERICANS CONNECTED WITH THIS BOOK) WITH YOUR BODIES.

3 SLOWLY, GO DOWN INTO A DEEP KNEE BEND AND SLOWLY RETURN TO YOUR ORIGINAL POSITION.

119

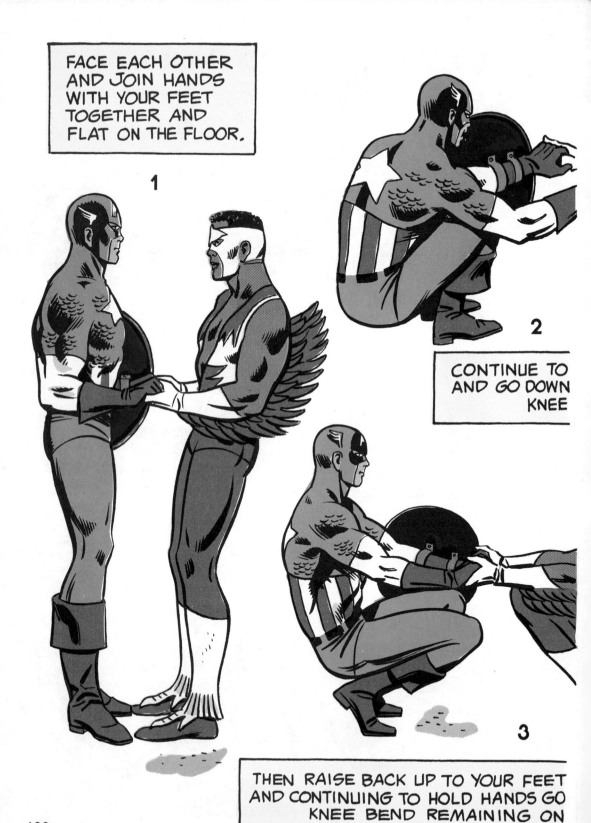

FACE EACH OTHER
AND JOIN HANDS
WITH YOUR FEET
TOGETHER AND
FLAT ON THE FLOOR.

1

2

CONTINUE TO
AND GO DOWN
KNEE

3

THEN RAISE BACK UP TO YOUR FEET
AND CONTINUING TO HOLD HANDS GO
KNEE BEND REMAINING ON

The Partnership's Patella Phlexers

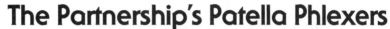

(ALL RIGHT, WE *KNOW* IT'S REALLY "FLEXER" BUT WE NEEDED ANOTHER "P" WORD).

HOLD HANDS INTO A DEEP BEND.

4

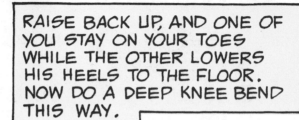

RAISE BACK UP, AND ONE OF YOU STAY ON YOUR TOES WHILE THE OTHER LOWERS HIS HEELS TO THE FLOOR. NOW DO A DEEP KNEE BEND THIS WAY.

LIFT UP TO YOUR TOES DOWN INTO ANOTHER YOUR TOES.

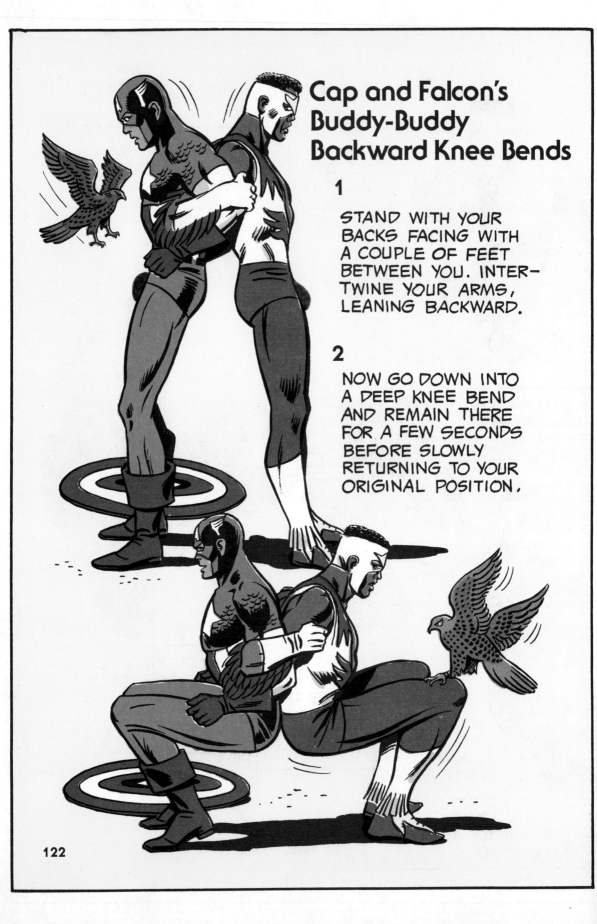

Cap and Falcon's Buddy-Buddy Backward Knee Bends

1

STAND WITH YOUR BACKS FACING WITH A COUPLE OF FEET BETWEEN YOU. INTER-TWINE YOUR ARMS, LEANING BACKWARD.

2

NOW GO DOWN INTO A DEEP KNEE BEND AND REMAIN THERE FOR A FEW SECONDS BEFORE SLOWLY RETURNING TO YOUR ORIGINAL POSITION.

THE FAMILY THAT PLAYS TOGETHER:

Things to Do with Family Members Other than Bicker

Firm in the belief that all work and no play makes Peter Parker a dull person, we now present a few little diversions designed by very clever and sadistic people to fool you into thinking exercise is fun.

If you already know any of these activities, let this section serve as a reminder that just because it's exercise doesn't necessarily mean you'll hate it. These are things you can do with your dad, brother or sister (or sibling) or even your mom. It's great exercise, and it sure beats playing Go Fish.

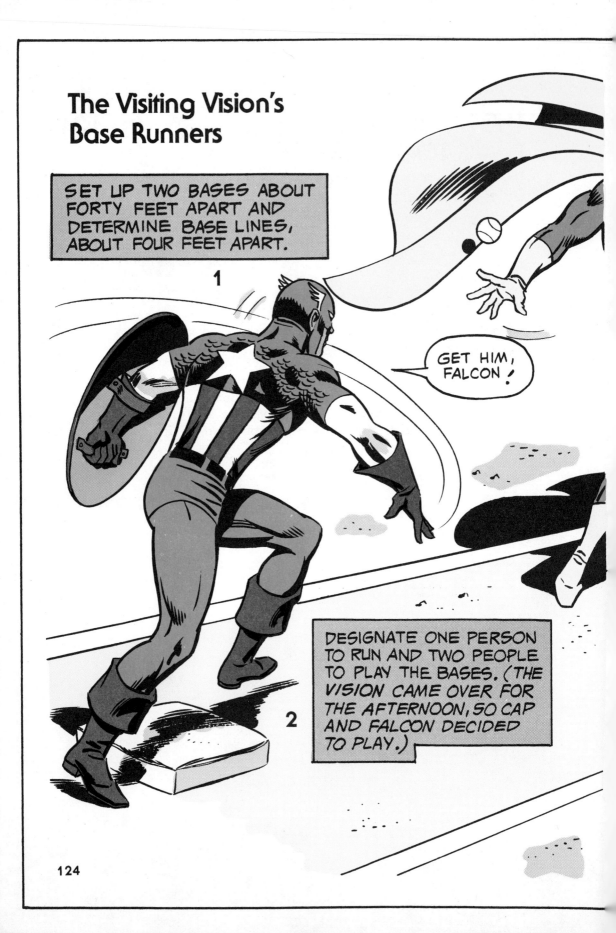

The Visiting Vision's Base Runners

SET UP TWO BASES ABOUT FORTY FEET APART AND DETERMINE BASE LINES, ABOUT FOUR FEET APART.

1

GET HIM, FALCON!

DESIGNATE ONE PERSON TO RUN AND TWO PEOPLE TO PLAY THE BASES. (THE VISION CAME OVER FOR THE AFTERNOON, SO CAP AND FALCON DECIDED TO PLAY.)

2

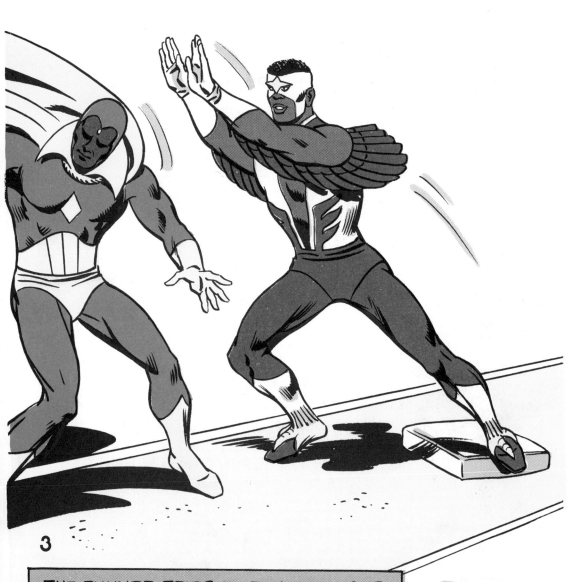

3

THE RUNNER TRIES TO RUN FROM ONE
BASE TO ANOTHER WITHIN THE BASE
LINES WITHOUT GETTING TAGGED OUT.

4

THE RUNNER SEES HOW MANY POINTS
HE CAN AMASS (OR MAKE, IF YOU WANT
TO KEEP IT SIMPLE) BEFORE GETTING
THREE OUTS.

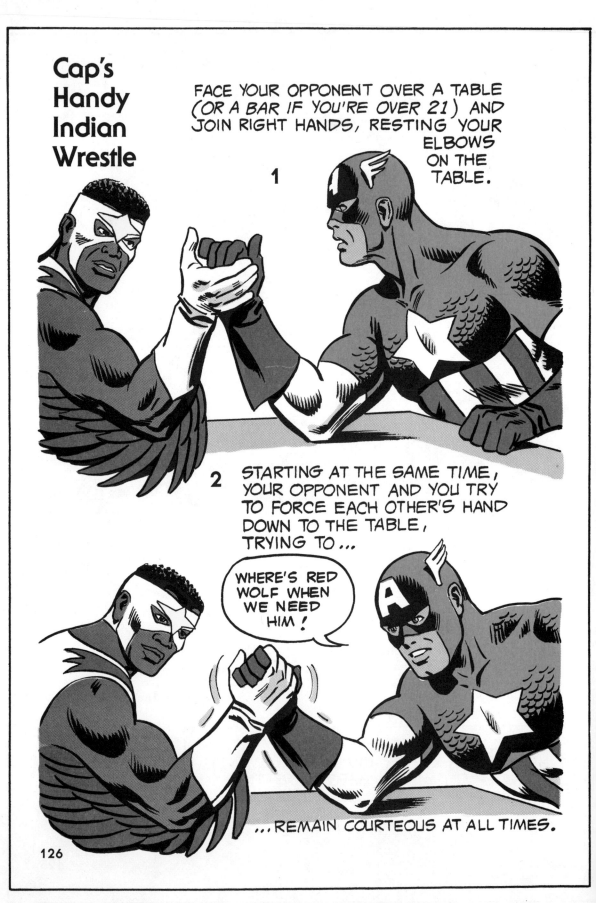

Cap's Not-So-Handy Indian Wrestle

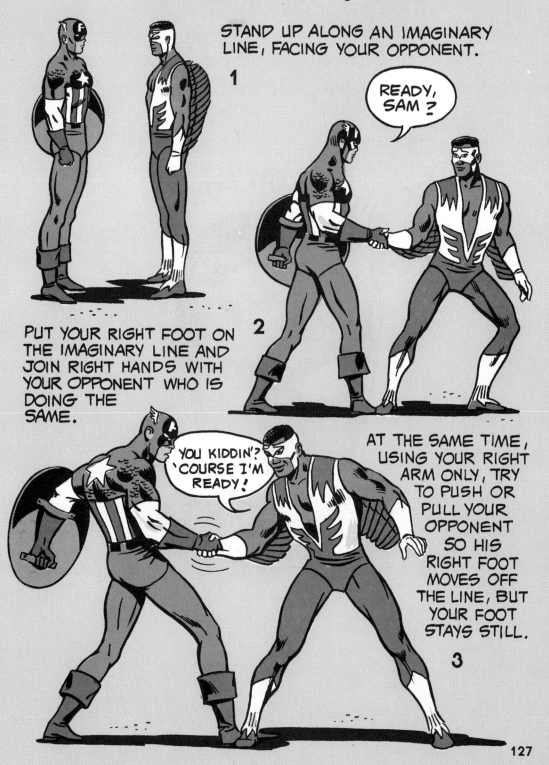

STAND UP ALONG AN IMAGINARY LINE, FACING YOUR OPPONENT.

1

READY, SAM?

PUT YOUR RIGHT FOOT ON THE IMAGINARY LINE AND JOIN RIGHT HANDS WITH YOUR OPPONENT WHO IS DOING THE SAME.

2

YOU KIDDIN'? 'COURSE I'M READY!

AT THE SAME TIME, USING YOUR RIGHT ARM ONLY, TRY TO PUSH OR PULL YOUR OPPONENT SO HIS RIGHT FOOT MOVES OFF THE LINE, BUT YOUR FOOT STAYS STILL.

3

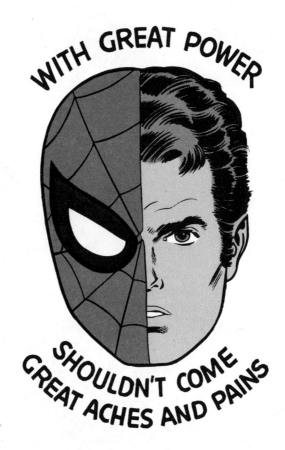